GROUPS

A Manual For Chemical Dependency and Psychiatric Treatment

John Olesen
Joanne Fallon
Louise Mark

CL Productions
Santa Fe, NM
1-800-203-3597

ISBN 1-887398-00-7

TABLE OF CONTENTS

Notes On Group Counseling 1
Group Counseling for Clients 7
Therapeutic Techniques 13

MEDICAL GROUPS

Disease Concept

Introduction 21
Disease Concept Lecture 23
Disease Concept Overview 41
Disease Concept Lecture Follow-Up 45
More On The Causes Of Alcoholism (Genetics & Environment) 49
Genetics Of Alcoholism: Family Tree 55

Medical Aspects Of Alcoholism

Introduction 59
Medical Aspects Lecture 63
Medical Lecture Follow-Up Groups 71
Trouble Shooting, Working With Denial 77
Twenty Questions 81
Denial 85
Food: The Mind Altering Drug 91
Caffeine: The Favorite Amphetamine 101
AIDS and Chemical Dependency 109
Guidelines To Working The Steps 121
Step 1 Workbook 123
Step 2 Workbook 155
Step 3 Workbook 163

THERAPY GROUPS

Check In 167
Assertiveness
Assertiveness Training 171
Assertiveness In Action 179
Boundaries
Understanding Boundaries 187
Physical And Emotional Boundaries 195
Sexuality 203
Affirmations 209
Listening 213
Mirror Exercise 217
Tools of Sobriety 221

Unfinished Business 225
Anger 227
The Missing Link 237
Grief and Loss 243
Suffering 249
Spirituality 253
To Change or Not to Change 257
Expectation Trap 261
Peer Group - Tough Love 265
Social Atoms 271
Three Chair Exercise 275
Honesty 277
Life Line 281
The Road Map to Recovery 285
Alcoholics Anonymous:
  AA: Questions, Questions, Questions 291
  Speaking In AA 297
  Things that Bug Me About AA 301

CODEPENDENCY AND FAMILY GROUPS
Introduction To The Groups 303
Codependency
  Codependency: Disease Concept 305
  Codependent Behaviors 321
Dysfunctional Families 329
About Blame 337
Family Roles 341
Abuse
  Abuse Lecture 349
  The Abuse Triangle 361
Multiple Family Group 367

RELAPSE AND RELAPSE PREVENTION
Relapse: Notes to Clinicians 371
The Developmental Process of Recovery 373
Relapse Happens Before It Happens 381
Relapse Prevention Plan 385
Recovery Plan Outline 393
Recovery Plan 399

Bibliography 405

INTRODUCTION

This manual is written to assist treatment programs by providing a resource of essential educational tools for the provision of chemical dependency treatment. Bonding and identification among chemically dependent clients is crucial to successful recovery, making "group treatment" the most effective modality. The ideas are not new and the content and formats of these groups will be familiar. Our goal is to provide a consolidated reference using information from a variety of sources and modalities.

The manual is presented sequentially, accommodating treatment stages and assimilation, with one group building and reinforcing the one before. It integrates the essential components of treatment, facilitating cognitive and experiential learning. **Groups** provides education, experiential reinforcement, fun and physical and emotional safety.

This manual can also assist in providing more consistent programming and a clear theoretical framework for treatment staff. Staff turnover in this field is high and training can be a tedious task for both supervisor and new employee. These simple groups introduce the newcomer to the field with a clear direction and enables them to begin facilitating groups early in training. It provides the same benefits to program interns and work study students. For veteran clinicians, our hope is that these groups will add new dimensions to your work and be fun for you, too.

GROUPS IN THE PSYCHIATRIC SETTING

Nearly all of the groups can be modified for family or psychiatric groups by substituting "AA" with "Al-Anon", or "alcoholism" with "depression" and so forth. You may need to alter the handouts to suit your treatment needs.

Here are a few examples of psychiatric or family groups:

codependency	assertiveness	anger
abuse	dysfunctional families	suffering
change	affirmations	sexuality
grief and loss	AIDS	family roles
boundaries	mirror exercise	defenses
listening	expectation trap	unfinished business

FOR DUAL DIAGNOSIS CLIENTS

Obviously, clients who suffer from major mental illnesses with psychotic components need to be recompensated and stabilized. Our groups are pertinent for all **stabilized** dual diagnosis clients. Depending upon the functioning level of the clients, modifications to the groups and lectures may or may not be needed.

For low functioning clients, breaking the groups into smaller pieces over time is suggested. In addition, adding action methods or incorporating styles described in "Therapeutic Techniques" is helpful to concretize the more conceptual lectures or groups. For example, diet is believed to be important for schizophrenics, eliminating sugars. When presenting the "Food" Lecture to schizophrenics, ask those who ate a little sugar that day to stand in one group, those who ate a lot to stand in another, etc. Have each person make a statement about how the sugar affected them, etc. As you initially review the groups to yourself, make notes about how to reframe the groups to meet your clients' needs.

For those clients with personality disorders, please keep in mind that you are seeing them clinically because the parts of their personalities which have been able to cope with their lives aren't functioning or able to integrate new stressors. They have decompensated. We generally see them when they are highly fragmented. As they lack healthy integration to begin with, we see them when their protective defenses are down and their underlying primitive feelings are surfacing and being painfully or overwhelmingly experienced by the client. Because they have disrupted identity formations, it is vital that the clinician avoid negative feedback as this will reinjure the wounded client or evoke rage to defend against it. These are very hard but workable clients. Again, utilizing the techniques and reframing the groups will be helpful. For help understanding these clients, we suggest reading "Humanizing The Narcissistic Style" by Stephen M. Johnson, PhD. It's published by W.W. Norton & Co., 1987, ISBN # 0-393-70037-2. Any and all books by Alice Miller are also highly recommended.

For more information about action methods and their application, review "Acting-In" by Adam Blatner, MD, Springer Publishing Co., and "Psychodrama, It's Application to ACOA and Substance Abuse Treatment", by Robert I. Fuhlrodt, ASCW. It can be ordered by calling the "Promise Bookstore", 1-201-403-1880.

NOTES ON GROUP COUNSELING

The group is an especially potent place in which to do counseling. For most clients, positive behavioral change occurs more quickly in a group. Yet, not everyone can or should lead a counseling group. Ethically, specific group counselor knowledge and skills must be met in order to be effective with clients. Becoming an expert in leading counseling groups is a professional development goal of great magnitude. As professionals, we must constantly seek to refine our skills and knowledge and to increase our repertoire of techniques and strategies for group counseling work. We encourage you to read, attend workshops, join professional counselor organizations, and align yourselves with experienced and skillful counselors.

Competency in group counseling often means introducing new structures, being creative, spontaneous and imaginative. Just as our clients are on a recovery journey, we, too, as counselors are on a magnificent road. We encourage you to develop your own strategies and apply your own new twists to those you pick up from us or other professionals.

We have found that there are some constantly recurring situations and times in counseling groups when an appropriate intervention is called for. Of course, immediate counselor intervention is called for on issues concerning the safety of an individual client or the group as a whole.

In other circumstances, we encourage the group to confront each other on their behaviors. We do this in the introduction to group counseling by giving permission and encouragement to the clients.

"This is your group. It is your responsibility to your own recovery to speak up about what you see, hear and feel about what is going on here. It is your work as a group member. No work, no payoff." During the course of the group, we might state, *"Bob, what did you hear or see happening when Susan was sharing about her financial difficulties?"*

As in the "Assertiveness: Into Action Presentation", we encourage the feedback form:

"When you___________, I feel________."

or

"When you said________, I felt________."

This helps clients to identify behaviors and feelings while discouraging advice giving or shaming.

Feelings are important in group work. They are not, however, the measure of success for the client or the group. Feelings are quite impossible without thoughts. Group counseling needs to address individual growth and the elimination of self-defeating behaviors. Too often, we see counselors whose only intervention is, *"And, how do you feel about that?"* They judge their competency by how much *"feeling"* was elicited in the group. For many newly recovering alcoholics and addicts having sober feelings is a new experience. We reinforce the idea that while we are fully responsible for our behaviors, *"we are powerless over our feelings."* To try and control or edit feelings is self-defeating for individual group work. Women get angry. Men cry and feel sad or scared. A major task for the leader and the entire group is to identify, to clarify, to label, and to reflect feelings. Any and all feeling is encouraged in group.

Certainly, any and all behavior is not.

The group counselor can serve as a model to the group members and actually teach them leadership intervention behaviors.

We have composed a list of often seen occasions which require intervention. This is by no means all-inclusive. In fact, one of the most exciting and challenging aspects of leading group counseling is that each group is different and every client has a unique contribution. Each person's perceptions are at least a shade different from every one else's.

Intervene if:

1. **A group member speaks for everyone.** For example: Bob, *"This group is a waste of time. We're not going anywhere. We are all wasting our time here."*

   This inhibits individual members from challenging each other for fear of going against the group.

   An appropriate intervention might include: *"You mentioned we, Bob. I hear you speaking for each person in the group. Is there anyone who doesn't agree?"*

   Another intervention might include going directly to another member, *"Jane, is Bob speaking for you?"*

   Bob's message is important. The group leader might simply redirect the client, *"Bob, I hear and see your frustration. Re-state what you just said as an "I" statement. What is going on for you, Bob, right now?*

2. **Self definitions**. A client states that *"I've always been that way."*
   For example: Sally, ***"Look, I'm shy.*** *That's just the way I am and I can't help it."*

A tendency of group members is to bring self-descriptions into their consciousness when they want an excuse for not working hard at changing. The self definition here is the statement *"I am a shy person"*.

The group counselor has the responsibility for seeing that the group helps each member deal effectively with the areas of her/his thinking which inhibit growth. Believing that the past dictates one's future is false and encourages people to function at lower levels than what they could attain.

An appropriate intervention might be to encourage feedback from other group members, *"Is there anyone else here who identifies with being shy? And, what are you doing about it?"*

Another intervention might be, *"Sally, the work of changing is very hard. I see your shyness holding you back. What does that feel like?"*

Many times clients will be overpowered by their own self-definitions. Change can be made in many tiny actions rather than by a single sweeping all-inclusive one. *"Sally, I hear you say how shy you are. And, still, you're speaking up in group. That's a lot for a shy person. When did you first notice your shyness? How has it held you back in the past?"*

3. **The non-participant.** Group leader, *"Jerry, we haven't heard from you in the last several sessions. And you haven't given any feedback to your peers, what's going on?"* Jerry, *"Nothing"* or *"I think I just need to listen. I'm getting a lot by just listening."*

   Individual progress can be impeded by other members who are simply "on for the ride." Certainly, by just listening, Jerry's recovery issues are not being addressed directly.

   One possible intervention might be, *"Jerry, when we don't let other people know who we are, they will invent us. You deserve more than that. The group can't address your specific recovery issues if you don't open up. What do you see as your primary recovery issue?"*

   Another intervention is to open it up to the group, *"How many of you think it is important for Jerry to take some group time? Can you help him out?"*

   In this intervention, as well as the others, the leader's sensitivity to the client's possible emotional state will be a key to the intervention. What is Jerry's body language, affect, and other group behavior telling you? He might be holding back because he is feeling bored, indifferent, insecure, angry, timid, or superior.

4. **Discrepancies.** It is crucial to effective group interaction that the leader see what is going on and name it. Trust-building is based on honest, open confrontation.

Warm, accepting approval of everything a client says and does creates a firm barrier to growth and will eventually disintegrate the group. Group members are not on trial, however, and anger and hostility from the group leader is a true disservice. The group needs to be a setting in which being plain and simple is a way of life. In group counseling the individual learns how to be direct and unabashedly candid in dealing with himself.

The intervention with discrepant behavior is to simply point out what you, as the leader, see going on. Care is taken not to prove the client "wrong" or shame him.

Many times there is a discrepancy between what a client is saying and what he/she said earlier. At other times there will be a difference between what a client is saying and doing. The group counselor must be willing to point out the gaps.

A common discrepancy is between what a client says and what he/she feels. Here the intervention comes with describing how the client's nonverbal behavior contradicts the content of the message. For example: *"Janet, I hear you say that everything is okay and that you're doing well. But, I need to tell you that your eyes look very, very sad and that there is a catch in your voice. Are you aware of this?"*

A fourth discrepancy is between what a client says about herself and how others in the group have been seeing her based on information that they have garnered at one time or another. Noticing reactions of the other group members when a client is taking time in the group can give the leader clarification as to how that person is seen. Sometimes it feels as if the group leader is always the last to know what is going on among the clients. Nonetheless, the question remains, *"What is going on?"* The question may be asked to the sharing client, to specific group members or to the group as a whole. It is important for the individual and for the group that it be asked.

With time, counselors will develop their intuitive sense about client discrepancies. Although we can often be off by assuming that our own reactive feelings point to a discrepancy, checking it out helps a client clarify where the psychological truth lies.

5. **The detached client. A client says,** *"It's not really my business to give Bill feedback. Besides, I don't want to hurt his feelings."* Clearly, an intervention is called for. In the early stages of a counseling group, clients often have the tendency to direct their responses or sharing to the leader alone. They will often expect you to do the group's work. The group leader is a facilitating guide and healthy groups are marked by client interaction. An appropriate intervention might be, *"Bill seems fairly hardy and strong to me. Ask him if he would like to hear your feedback."* Pointing out reasons for the fear of being forthright will encourage clients to share perceptions and feelings which they see will contribute to the welfare of another member. A lifeboat where each person keeps to himself will never make it to

shore. If, on the other hand, the people in the lifeboat work together, everyone has a chance.

6. **Aggressive behavior in group.** Any kind of aggressive behavior in group, either physical or verbal, is not to be tolerated. It may be as innocuous as interrupting. The leader must immediately confront that person and stop the action. After a beat, the leader should restate the ground rules for the group and contract with the aggressive person and the group. Anger and aggression build. The earlier the leader intervenes, the less dramatic the confrontation. Besides creating safety for the clients, you are responsible for your own well-being.

7. **The client who plays counselor.** Many times clients will try to help their peers by imitating a therapist. Usually, they are seeking approval from the group or group leader. Other times, these questions and statements are overt passive/aggressive behavior. Often heard client techniques include:

   A. Making stereotypical comments. For example: *"Keep your chin up. It's not that bad."*

   B. Giving literal responses. For example: Client A., *"I feel like getting a gun."* Client B., *"Oh, really? What kind of gun?"*

   C. Interpreting. For example: *"What you really mean is . . ."*

   D. Rejecting. For example: *"I don't want to hear about that again."*

   E. Judging. For example: *"Now that is really disgusting."*

   F. Abruptly changing the subject. For example: Client A., *"I'm feeling sad today."* Client B., *"By the way, where did you buy your shoes?"*

   An intervention with a light touch can keep clients from feeling shamed and get the group back on course. Remember, these clients are often seeking approval and, in general, most of the people in the group will have very low self-esteem. An appropriate intervention at this point might be, *"Jim, it's great you're jumping in with feedback. Remember to stick with what you see and what you hear. And then, how you feel about that. Give it another try. Without any interpretation, what do you hear Sarah saying?"*

8. **Externally focused.** A client who focuses on people, conditions, or events outside the group. For example: *"My wife is the reason I drink. She depresses me and I drink when I am depressed."*

   Alcoholism and addiction are outwardly focused diseases. Counseling groups can easily turn into gripe sessions without early intervention. Many times clients

> will reinforce and support each other's attitudes about how the world (or the people in it) tend to conspire unfairly against them. A feeling of common solidarity can prop them up in their apparently common struggle. Frequently bashed targets include, wives, husbands, men, women, parents, children, employers, counselors. An appropriate intervention might be, *"Dave, you keep mentioning your wife as the source of your being depressed. I think it is more important to look at yourself. What is your part in the dynamic?"* This might also be an excellent place to point out a discrepancy, *"Dave, I hear you say your wife is the reason you drink. I want to point out, however, that you told me in your assessment that you were drinking heavily 10 years before you met her."*

Any intervention needs to focus clients back to themselves. Talking about "them or they" in the group can do nothing but reinforce a client's mentality of believing someone else is to blame.

These are but eight occasions necessitating intervention. There are many more. Processing what went on in the group with a co-leader is an excellent way to improve your intervention techniques. Keeping group records and notes of the interactions is another. The interventions we have shown here are quite basic. With experience comes an increase in the comfortability, creativity, and respect that the group leader brings to the group.

GROUP COUNSELING FOR THE CLIENTS

This presentation outlines the purpose of group counseling and lets clients know what is expected of them in group. Present this group on an on-going basis as new members enter the group. Frequent review of the group counseling guidelines and handouts is essential for maintaining an active group. The more familiar the clients are with the group goals and guidelines, the greater the safety they will feel. Repetition, repetition, repetition. We ask for peer explanations from "older" clients as much as possible.

We strongly recommend reviewing group expectations and goals frequently.

What Is Group Counseling?

Group is a safe place to talk about what is going on in your recovery. In group we share thoughts, memories, and feelings. The group can give you insight, support, and acceptance. It is a safe place to take the risk to open up to others. It is a safe place to dare to care and support your peers.

What is expected?

What is said in group, stays in group. You may share your own issues with anyone you choose. It is **not** acceptable to talk about group interaction or other peoples' issues outside the group. The staff, however, may share group information with each other in professional meetings in order to better serve you and make your treatment plan more specific.

There are **two** circumstances where information will not be kept in this room. These are the **only** two. As therapists we are legally bound to disclose:

1. If you are physically, emotionally, or sexually abusing a child.
2. If you are planning to kill or physically harm yourself or someone else.

Honesty is the key to opening up. True self-expression is the fastest way to make contact with others. We don't have to express ourselves perfectly. Group is the place to honestly talk about what is difficult, hard to say, puzzling, hurtful, or troubling.

Listen to everyone. Make sure that everyone is listened to. In group, we listen with our ears, our eyes, and our feelings. Try to sense the living and feeling part of each group member and respect the feelings being expressed.

Give feedback. Group members are expected to share what they see and hear going on with the other members of the group. This means sharing feelings as well. One format we have found to be particularly helpful is: State what you see or hear, and then, what you feel.

*"**When you**________, **I feel**________."*

An example is: *"Bill, **I see you opening up** and talking about what is going on at home. And last week, you said everything was fine. **When you** are really honest like this, **I feel** hopeful for you."*

No pretending. Just by being in group, you do not stop being the person you are on the outside. If things are going on between you and someone else outside of the group, don't pretend the conflict doesn't exist. It does. In group, the masks and games are left behind.

This is your group. Group members are expected to confront group interaction and help it grow to become an ever more powerful tool for achieving personal change. This means that group members will initiate discussions about barriers which exist in the group, communication problems, and problems of group unity and trust.

The more you put in, the more you'll take out. Group is a place for active participation. It will not serve you or others to merely take up space. All of us know how scary it can be to risk opening up and letting others really see us. That is why we ask "new" people to jump in on their first group and simply tell the other group members something about who they are and what brings them to the group. At your last group, we will ask you to take time for termination, to review what you received from the group and to share your plans and goals.

HANDOUT # 1

HOW TO GET THE MOST OUT OF GROUP

1. What goes on in the group is the property of the group. It stays in group.
2. Give feedback. (State what you see or hear and then, what you feel.)
3. Take "time". Focus on the issues you need to work on.
4. Participate as fully as possible. The more you put in, the more you'll take out.
5. Use "I" statements.
6. Keep an open mind. Be willing to discover positive and negative, growing and limiting sides of yourself.
7. See the group as a safe place for growth. Group is a place for progress, not perfection.
8. Use the group to practice new behaviors.
9. Think of ways to apply what you are learning in group to your life outside the group.
10. Pay attention to your own body language and feelings. Don't shut them out.
11. Leave masks and games outside the group.
12. Avoid postponing the risk taking involved in letting others know you.
13. You "earned" your seat in group. Don't apologize for your statements.
14. Remember, changes take time and effort.

HANDOUT # 2

COMMON GROUP BEHAVIORS

Here is a list of frequently seen group behaviors that need to be confronted as they happen. Take the risk to confront your own behavior. Take the risk to confront the behaviors of your peers. Whether they are directly connected to drinking/using or not, these behaviors will lead to relapse.

1. **Excuse Making** — For example: *"I drink because I'm depressed"* or *"I drink because my wife doesn't understand me."*

2. **Blaming** — Blaming permits the build-up of resentments and gets the focus off the alcoholic and puts it on others. For example: *"The trouble with you is that you always you're so critical. Who wouldn't drink!"*

3. **Redefining** — Shifts the focus of an issue to avoid solving the problem. For example: Q: *"Why did you stop going to AA and go to the bar last night?"* A: *"I feel that the language in the "Big Book" is old fashioned and too religious."*

4. **Super-Optimism** — For example: *"I think, therefore, it is." "I can stop drinking because I put my mind to it. I don't need any support."*

5. **Lying** — Confuses, distorts and takes the focus off the behavior. Examples are:
   Commission - making things up that are simply not true.
   Omission - leaving out major sections.
   Assent - presenting others' ideas to look good with no intention of following through.

6. **Making Fools of Others** — By putting others down, we take the focus off our own behaviors.

7. **Assuming** — For example: *"Nobody cares about me anyway."* Gives us an excuse to blow up, get angry or get drunk.

8. **I'm Unique** — *"No one can tell me what to do."*

9. **Ingratiating** — Finding out what you can get from other people, how you can control them, use them or control the situation for your own purposes. For example: *"You're my favorite counselor."*

10. **Minimizing** — For example: *"I only drank three beers."*

11. **Vagueness** — Being unclear and nonspecific to avoid being pinned down. *"I guess", "Probably", "Maybe", "I'm not sure about this", "I drink socially", "I smoke pot occasionally"*, and *"I've used it"*.

12. **Aggression**— Scaring others by our power and strength so that they will agree with us or leave us alone.

13. **Power Plays**— Walking out of a room during a disagreement or organizing others to support our anger.

14. **Victim Playing** — Acting like the King Baby, or whining and acting helpless, and acting too stupid to do anything for ourselves.

15. **Drama/Excitement**— A distraction which keeps the focus off our own behavior.

16. **Secretive and Close Minded** — Opposite of going to any length of whatever works.

17. **Image and Self-Definition** — For example: *"That's me. That's just the way I am. I'm just a quiet person"*.

18. **Grandiosity** — For example: *"I've spilled more booze than you've drank."*

19. **Intellectualizing** — Using academic, abstract, or theoretical discussions to avoid dealing with the feelings associated with the issue. *"My memory problems? Anybody who drinks for a long time will experience some cognitive deficits."*

20. **Staying in the Safety Zone** — Withholding information because of the fear of confrontation.

Remember, this is about behavior, not the person. We confront what we see another group member doing, not who he or she is. Just by being in group guarantees you unconditional respect as a person.

THERAPEUTIC TECHNIQUES

There are different techniques for working with clients who are either actively and openly resistant or in subconscious denial. While many of us have our different styles and therapeutic approaches, it's nice to have some simple techniques which can be shared among the staff. We have listed and explained some techniques which work well for us and can be easily utilized.

SCALING QUESTIONS

Scaling questions are ways to have your clients place themselves along a continuum of some of form of recovery. It assumes that life and behavior develop along a linear progression. Clients place themselves along the continuum and make decisions about moving forward or backward along whichever scale or stage fits their issues.
For example, suppose that the medical aspects of alcoholism are placed along a linear progression chart, from less severe symptoms to most severe symptoms.

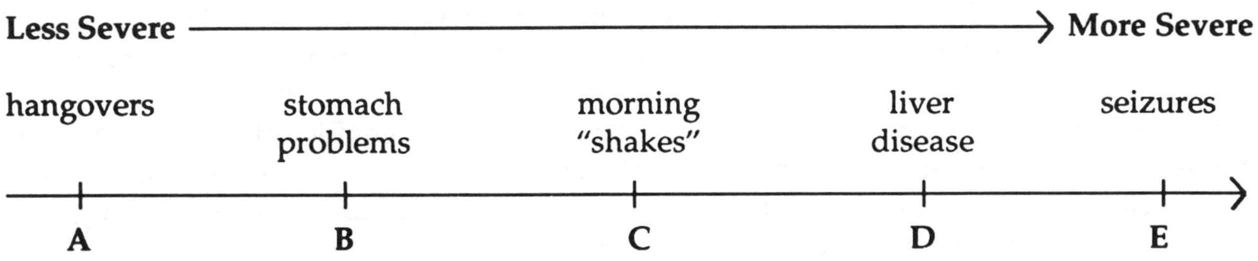

Suppose that your client, Tom, has experienced all of the symptoms from A through E, but is only able to self-identify up to point C. He has denial about D, liver disease and E, seizures, so he is not convinced that he is alcoholic. Direct confrontation does not get him to accept that he is really at point E. How can you get Tom to shift his position from C to E?

Show him the continuum.

Keep the initial stage of his work general, having him talk about a generic person. Have Tom identify at which place along the line he feels that **"somebody"** is **definitely** alcoholic (not necessarily him).

Tom identifies point E, seizures.
Ask Tom where he is on the scale.

Tom chooses point C, he's had "shakes" a few times.

The goal is to have Tom shift his beliefs about at which point "**somebody**" is **definitely** alcoholic. Since he chooses point E, the goal is to have him shift his beliefs from point E down to the next lowest notch, point D, liver disease.

Explain that we know that point D, liver disease, is caused by alcoholism and that there are stages of liver disease (a continuum). Show Tom the liver disease continuum.

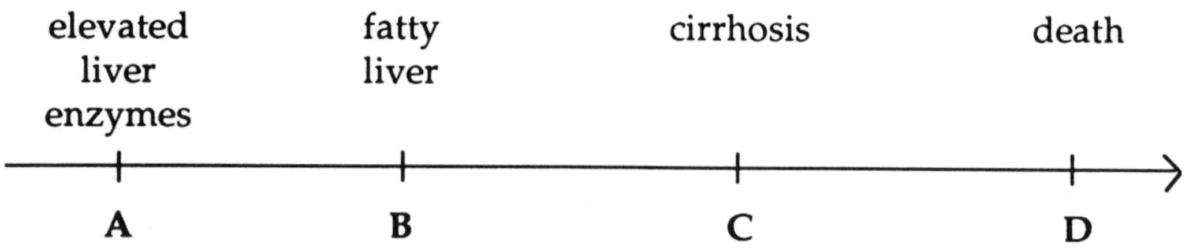

Have Tom identify at which point along **this** line, the liver disease continuum, somebody could be identified as alcoholic.

Tom says point C, cirrhosis.
Tom has just shifted his position. He has identified a symptom in point D as definitely alcoholic. From the first scale, he has moved from point E, seizures, to point D, cirrhosis.

This is the format of using this type of scaling question. The client identifies where they see themselves, on a continuum. The therapist has them identify themselves at the next position in that continuum. There are continuum within continuum. To keep working with Tom lay out the continuum about cirrhosis:

Example: "*Nobody wakes up one day with cirrhosis. Cirrhosis occurs over time. Liver disease has early and late stages. Cirrhosis is the very end stage of alcoholism and liver disease.* " Here are the stages:

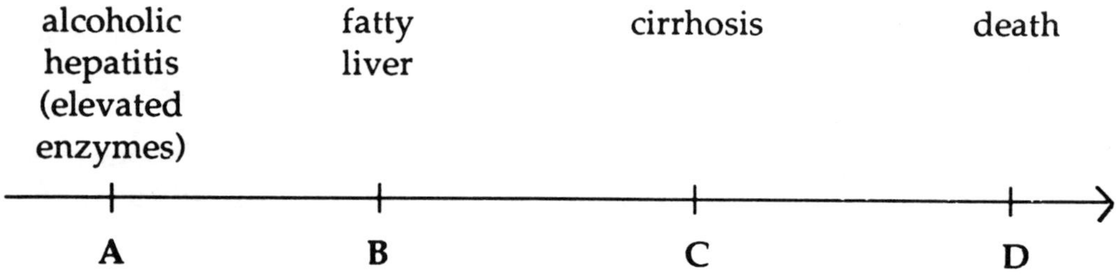

Therapist: "So Tom, at which point on this scale could we tell that Mr. X **will end up with** cirrhosis?"

Tom: *"Point B, fatty liver."*

Therapist: *"How will Mr. X know that he is at point B?"*

Tom: *"Blood tests?"*

Therapist: *"So what you're telling me Tom, is that if Mr. X has blood work that is abnormal, he can be fairly certain that he has got the disease of alcoholism. Is that correct?"*

If he says no, start at the beginning again. If he says yes, now personalize it to fit for Tom.

Therapist: *"Tom, you just told me that you think an alcoholic is a person with liver disease and that one way to tell is to look at their blood tests. Can we look at yours?"*
These are normal values, these are yours. What do you now know about your physical status?"

Because Tom, not the therapist, changed his position to define alcoholism, Tom has created his own reality by his definition. Tom has told you that 2 + 2 = 4, or fatty liver disease plus abnormal lab values = alcoholism.
Should Tom conclude that 2 + 2 = 5, start again. The goal with scaling questions is for the client to come to his own conclusion. **It is always more effective for the client to diagnose himself.** If the therapist states a fact, it is subject to question and challenge. If I state a fact, it must be true.

This type of scaling can be used for nearly any issue, to move the client from point A to point B. From rigid belief to less rigid beliefs, from rigid behavior to less rigid behavior, from denial to acceptance. Use it with your work on identifying dysfunctional families, abuse, acceptable behavior, etc.

Example: Tom doesn't feel that he is from a dysfunctional family.

Families are functional along a continuum. Some are very healthy, some beat their children to death. Draw in a continuum chart.

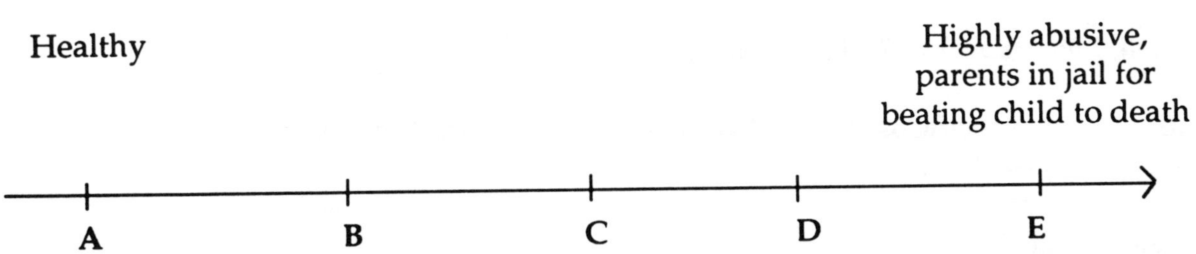

Numbered Scaling Questions

Another type of scaling question involves numbers.
"On a scale of 1 to 10, Where do you see yourself?"
"You are a four?"
"What would you need to do to be a five?"

These types of scaling questions work well for assessing where your client sees themself, and how to change their behavior to see themselves differently.

Example:

Client: *"I'm depressed."*

Therapist: *"On a scale of one to ten, with one being suicidal, can't get out of bed, can't think at all, can't eat, and 10 being exceptionally happy, the world is perfect, where do you see yourself?"*

Client: *"I'm a three."*

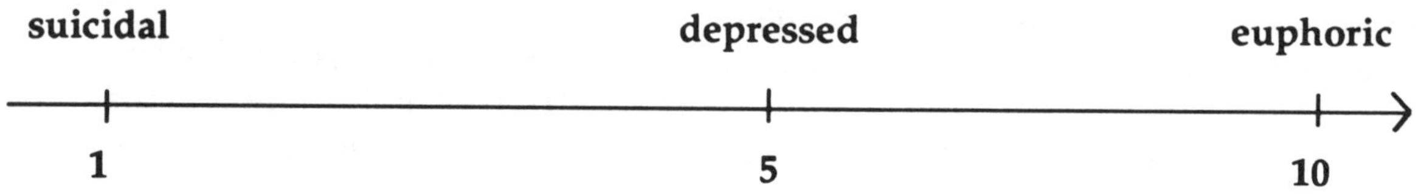

The goal is to have the person identify what they can do to be a four, the next number on the scale of emotional health.

Do not focus on the client as being a three!

Therapist: *"Have you ever felt like a four?"*

Client: *"A long time ago."*

Th: *"What things did you do differently when you were a four?"* (look for specific behaviors).

Cl: *"Well, I had more friends. I was going out more."*

Th: (identifying specific behavior) *"So you're telling me that if you call a friend and go out, you usually feel like a four."*

Cl: *"I suppose so."*

Th: *"It seems like you already know how to move yourself out of some your depression. What do you need to do when feel like a three and you want to feel like a four?"*

Cl: *"Call a friend."*

These numerical scaling questions work especially well with couples. The couple can rate themselves on a scale of one to ten (they say five). What is different when they're a six, i.e. **what different behavior does each person do individually to make the relationship a six?**

Therapist: *"Tom, what are you doing when the relationship is a six?"*
"Mary, what are you doing when the relationship is a six?"

If they want to be a six, he needs to do ________, she needs to do ________.

To be a two, he needs to do ________, she needs to do ___________.

When the person can identify specific behaviors which alter their mood and level of functioning, they have more power over choosing which behavior to increase.

The scaling questions are not intended to replace the need for ongoing therapy, but if incorporated as part of the therapy, can empower and motivate clients. Scaling questions help clients identify their destructive or self-destructive behaviors versus their healthy and ego strengthening behaviors. They are able to identify which behaviors they can increase to change their lives.

CHAIR WORK

Chair work can be a very powerful tool. One does not need to be a master clinician to reap the benefits of simple chair work. It is particularly useful for clients who are "stuck", can't separate issues, or can't formulate a plan for themselves. Chair work is useful in every clinical area because the client essentially tells themselves what the problem is, what to do, and how to do it.
The format is to place two chairs side by side.

The client makes a statement indicating that they are "stuck," indecisive or confused.
Example: *"I don't know if I can get sober."*

Directions: set up two chairs. Have the client sit in chair #1, the NOW chair.

Therapist: *"I want you to move over here and sit in this chair (#1) and tell me more about not knowing if you can stay sober."*

Client: *"I've tried before and never make it past two weeks. I have cravings all day long. I'm not sure I want to quit drinking."*

Th: (explore more about the statement until you are certain that you understand what they mean by their dilemma or problem.)
"I think I now understand what you mean. I'd like you to sit in chair #2, the future, after six months of sobriety. Tell me what is different about your life today."

Cl: *"I feel really healthy. My job is stable. I have more friends, I'm a lot happier."*

Th: *"You used to relapse after two weeks. How did you manage to stay sober all the time?"*

Cl: *"I'm not sure. I guess I went to AA meetings."*

Th: ***Repeat back specific behaviors.*** *"So going to AA helped. What is one more thing you did to help you stay sober?"*

Cl: *"I didn't call my old drinking friends."*

Th: *"So for you to stay sober and be happy,* ***you go to AA*** *and* ***don't see your old friends.*** *Would you share this with chair #1? She seems to be confused about what will help her."*

Direct the client to speak to the empty chair #1 and explain to it what she did to stay sober.
Thank the client, and ask her to return to chair #1.

Therapist: *"It sounds like you really know how to stay sober. It also sounds like* (indicate to the empty chair #2) *you like being sober and are able to do it. What directions do you hear yourself say which will keep you sober, or go* ***from chair #1 to chair #2?"***

Client: *"I need to go to AA and stay away from my using friends."*

After the client has identified the problem and solution, have them move back to the original chair from which they started the session. It is important for them to recognize that both of the voices belonged to them and have equal power and equal value.

Use analogies, such as chair #2 being their "Higher Self," or their "Inside, all knowing Self." Each person has the ability to identify personal solutions, they contain their own knowledge. Chair work allows them to experience this reality about themselves.

As mentioned, simple chair work can be used in any situation where there is conflict. It is also a powerful tool in group, where the "working" client can get feedback from the group on both "chairs".

THE FAIRY GODMOTHER TECHNIQUE:

This is a simple technique which uses the same concept as the scaling questions and chair work, however the approach is different. In this scenario, you are asking the client to describe "the perfect world" and to look at some practical behavioral changes they can make to move closer to it. It's another way to shift them from point A to point B.

This type of questioning is used for assessing children's abuse because it taps into their magical thinking and allows them more freedom to self-disclose. It also works well with adults who have the capacity to fantasize.

In this situation, tell the client that his fairy godmother has secretly waved her magic wand over his life and made everything perfect. Ask the client how he would know that the magic wand has been waved over his life. How can he tell that his life is now perfect? What is **different** today about himself,
his relationships,
his jobs?

There is an expression that *"God doesn't give us a dream without also giving us the capacity to make it come true."*

The follow up work with this fairy godmother question involves asking clients one or two things they can do today to create their dream.

How do they move from point A., today, to point E., the perfect world?
By going to point B.
What does **point B look like?**
What **actions** did they take to get to point B?

DISEASE CONCEPT INTRODUCTION

The Disease Concept lecture is the most important component of treatment. Like any other disease process, people can recover if they first understand what the disease is and how it affects their bodies. What makes chemical dependency difficult to treat is the social stigma associated with having the disease, compounded by the client's own negative myths and misinformation which they bring to treatment.

The challenge to clinicians is to provide a comprehensive medical overview of the disease which is thorough, up to date, non shaming, and objective. If this is acheived, our clients have the opportunity to begin their recovery with a fresh and optimistic outlook. They can then challenge their old belief systems about what it means to be chemically dependent.

Our concern in this section of the manual was how to provide the best materials for you to present to your clients. **The most outstanding presentations of the disease concept we have seen are lectures by David Ohlms M.D.**

The Gary Whiteaker Corporation has allowed us to provide you with Dr Ohlms' "The Disease Of Alcoholism" lecture. *It is the next group in this manual.* This lecture is also available to you to order as a pamphlet which can be used as patient handouts. **We strongly recommend utilizing the film "Addiction Disease" or "The Disease Of Alcoholism" in conjunction with the rest of the lectures. This is the most effective and comprehensive teaching method.** Please understand that we are not associated with their company nor benefit in any way should you decide to use their materials. Clients and families will greatly benefit from these wonderful videos. They are simply the best in the field.

To present the disease concept, we recommend using Dr. Ohlms' "Disease Of Alcoholism" lecture **in conjunction with the film.** In the "Disease Concept Overview" we have summarized some of the major points in the lecture. Once the disease concept has been reviewed with clients, we suggest using the rest of the presentations in the manual *in the order provided* to build on the material and begin to individualize treatment.

If you are a very small facility with a limited educational budget, GWC Inc. may be able to make some special arrangements for their videos, audio tapes, and books. They are open to discussion if you describe your circumstances to them.

To review the videos, contact: Gary Whiteaker Corporation
P.O. Box 5023
Cahokia, IL 62206
1-800-851-5406

The Disease Of Alcoholism

By David Ohlms, M.D.

Provided by: The Gary Whiteaker Corporation
(1-800-851-5406)

Much recent news from medical science seems to be discouraging: all kinds of everyday things have been found to cause cancer, heart disease, lung disease. There are even deadly diseases turning up that we hadn't heard of a few years ago. But there is good news about one of mankind's oldest diseases - alcoholism. Not too many years ago nearly everybody thought it was hopeless. We don't think so anymore.

I suppose the first part of the news is that alcoholism is a disease, a true disease, like cancer or diabetes or high blood pressure. It probably sounds strange to call that "good" news. But I can show you why it is good. And to do that, I have to tell you a story.

AA LEADS THE WAY

The story begins in the late 1930's when people who were suffering and dying from alcoholism got tired of going to professionals (physicians, psychiatrists, psychologists) because the professionals couldn't seem to help them - the alcoholics just kept on dying. Or wound up in lunatic asylums or jails. So alcoholics banded together and formed an organization to help themselves - Alcoholics Anonymous - and lo and behold, they did discover a way to stop dying and make themselves better.

AA members not only stopped dying and got healthier: they discovered a method that let them give up drinking and lead as normal a life as anyone else. That's the second part of the good news. But in order to help fellow alcoholics, AA first had to decide that alcoholism was a treatable disease. Let's go back to that half of the good news now.

This is my favorite part of the story. You have to remember that early AA members weren't medical research scientists - they were businessmen, salesmen, carpenters, waitresses - and they were all seemingly hopeless drunks who only recently had been able to stop drinking. But the AA Program was so successful that finally, after several decades, medical science felt forced to take a good look at it. Why did it work? Why was it that these ordinary people, doing what they did, were able to get well, while we professionals, treating them medically and psychiatrically, seemed to make them sicker rather than better?

The first thing we noticed was that Alcoholics Anonymous people were saying that alcoholism is a primary disease. It is its own disease. It causes its own symptoms - it is not itself a symptom of some other disease - and AA treated it this way. And medical science finally had to admit that AA was right! In 1956 the American Medical Association officially recognized Alcoholism as a true disease - an entity of and by itself, that created its own problems, its own symptoms, that had its own treatment - and the AMA published this view in a major paper.

This turned a lot of things around. It led to legislation that required a hospital to admit alcoholic patients, whereas before they hadn't wanted anything to do with those "drunks". Before 1956, doctors would often have to fix alcoholics up with a phony diagnosis in order to get them hospitalized at all. And then alcoholic patients would often be treated for secondary illnesses - liver disease, for example - while their major problem was ignored. So patients would go home with slightly improved livers - and completely unimproved alcoholism which soon wrecked their livers all over again! But since 1956 treatment centers have been opened throughout the United States, and indeed throughout the world, where people can go and get decent and humane care for their alcoholism

TRIPPING OVER DEFINITIONS

Now in order to go on with our story, we need to say something here about *disease*. I think we need to define it, and that's not easy to do. When I went to one of the very expensive medical dictionaries that I struggled to buy in medical school, it said that "disease is an illness". Very useful. When I looked up "illness" it defined illness as a "disease". I threw the book away and went and got a 99 cent pocket dictionary at a bookstore, and it had something I really liked. It defined disease as **anything that interferes with the ability of the human being to function normally.** That may be an infection such as tuberculosis, which can destroy your lungs. It may be the broken leg you got while pushing you car on an icy road. Whatever it is, however you caught it, a disease prevents you from living your life as efficiently as you ordinarily would.

Alcoholism clearly interferes with normal life more than any other disease. Few other primary diseases produce the range of emotional and physical complications caused by addiction to the drug alcohol. Not only is alcoholism destructive to practically every organ system in the human body, it erodes self-esteem, produces depression, promotes violence and destroys relationships.

American society is ambivalent and confused about the use of the drug alcohol, and those with alcoholism suffer all the more because of it. The predominate message of our culture, reinforced by slick advertising and other media images, is that everyone should be able to drink without losing control reinforces the opinion that there is something very wrong with the basic character of those who do lose control. This is why those who suffer from the disease of alcoholism have historically been referred to in derisive terms: wino, lush, drunks, boozers, etc.

The coming years will see a change in these attitudes. In fact, society is showing signs of general recognition of alcoholism as a *real* disease. This is happening because ongoing social and medical research is producing more and more evidence that alcoholism has a physical basis, and that out-of-control drinking is caused by inherited or developed quirks in the brain chemistry.

These neurochemical quirks can and do occur in sinners, saints, and everyone in between. This would explain why AA meetings, treatment centers and hospitals are filled with people from all walks of life and all socio/economic/ educational/religious backgrounds.

We'll start with the definition of the disease published by the American Medical Association:

Alcoholism is an illness characterized by : *preoccupation with alcohol; by loss of control over its consumption, such as to usually lead to intoxication or drinking done by chronicity; by progression and by tendency to relapse. It is typically associated with physical disability and impaired emotion, occupational and/or social adjustments as a direct consequence of persistent and effective use.*

Whew! Pretty wordy, isn't it?

For this reason, the AMA definition is not particularly good one. It's accurate, yes. Very valid, yes. But who could remember it if they really needed to?
Here is the definition I use and the one I prefer:

Alcoholism is a chronic, progressive, incurable disease characterized by loss of control over alcohol and other sedatives.

Now let me explain some of the major words in this much shorter definition.

Chronic is self explanatory. It lasts a long time.

Progressive is fascinating and the one most frustrating features of the illness. I want to carefully explain the progressive nature of alcoholism. Progressive simply means that alcoholism never gets any better -*even after a victim stops drinking!* Nearly all people who suffer from alcoholism have experienced the treachery of alcoholism's progressiveness. In fact, one of the key symptoms of alcoholism is repeated efforts to control drinking by "going on the wagon".

After a period of abstinence, the drinker attempts normal social drinking or reduced consumption. The result is always the same: the alcoholism returns full blown, as bad or worse, in a very short period of time.

Imagine the demoralizing impact this has had on victims of alcoholism and the people around them! Untreated alcoholism is a downward spiral of hope followed by despair followed by hope again followed by hopelessness. I would like to engrave a message in the minds of everyone in recovery from alcoholism: If you remain clean and dry, the coming months and years will bring remarkable and often miraculous improvements in your spiritual, emotional, physical, and social well being. But alcoholism is always waiting to be activated by a single drink! I have had many patients in recovery who have remained clean and dry for 5, 10, even 20 years, who have undergone remarkable improvements in physical and emotional health, who have restored good relationships with their families, employers, neighbors, and friends. One day they decided it was okay to take a drink. And incredibly, within days or weeks they were back on the horrendous merry-go-round of alcoholism, their lives crumbling around them. **It was as if they had never stopped drinking.**

ALCOHOLISM DOESN'T GO AWAY

Why? The answer in my opinion, is because alcoholism is a disease based on quirky metabolism and neurochemistry. The victim of alcoholism can, during periods of abstinence, change his or her attitudes through counseling and support groups and vastly improve physical health through regular exercise, good diet, sleep, etc., but they **cannot change the way they metabolize alcohol or their neurochemical response to the drug alcohol!.** We humans resist the idea of losing control over anything. But those who suffer from diabetes, heart disease, cancer, blindness, paralysis, and so on must sooner or later accept that they have little or no control over the physiological processes - the inherited or acquired physical abnormalities - which resulted in their condition. The same is true with alcoholism. But we started this book by saying there is good news about alcoholism. Alcoholism is one of the few chronic, progressive, fatal diseases that can be arrested and whose victims can live healthy, normal lives into a ripe old age!

IN PURSUIT OF DEFINITION

But let's go on with the definition. Alcoholism is an incurable disease - that to me is undeniable. We've already touched on this in the paragraphs above. Victims of the disease can return to normal life, but only for as long as drinking is stopped. You will come upon an occasional rare medical study that says differently - that says an alcoholic can be taught to handle controlled social drinking. If you are an alcoholic, ***don't believe it.***. Science has so far given us no cure for alcoholism.

Now we've said that alcoholism is a chronic, progressive incurable disease characterized by loss of control over alcohol and other sedatives. It is *characterized by loss of control*. That may sound so obvious as to be trivial but it is a very important medical definition . It's what makes this disease different from other chronic, incurable diseases such as diabetes and arthritis of some types. Loss of control does not mean, as many laymen and indeed professionals seem to think, that when an alcoholic takes a drink, every time he takes a drink - he's going to drink to excess and get drunk.

That's very rare. Alcoholics usually understand this far better than the professionals who treat them. Most of my patients tell me that there were times right before they landed in the hospital when they had a drink or two on a given occasion- and then stopped. They had no more alcohol that day. And if you would look at just that little 24 hour period, you would assume that such people were normal, controlled drinkers. But what *loss of control* means is that once the alcoholic takes that first drink after a period of being sober or abstinent, he can't predict with any reliability whether he's going to have a normal or abnormal drinking episode.

Look at it this way. On Monday, Uncle Jack gets off work at 5: he plans to stop by the Circle Tap Barroom, have a couple quick ones with colleagues, and then get home in time for supper. And he does exactly that. On Wednesday - it may have been a bad day, a good day, it doesn't seem to matter - Jack drops by the Circle Tap and has the same first couple of shots with the same colleagues and the very same intentions. The next thing he knows, the bar is closing. His friends are long gone. He climbs in his car, gets a drunk driving ticket or kills somebody on the way home; or, if he's lucky enough not to do that, he discovers, when he does get safely home, that the wife has packed her bags and left with the children.

Jack couldn't have told you that morning which way the day was going to go. The decision wasn't in his hands. He no longer controls alcohol, as most of us do; it controls him.

ALCOHOLISM = SEDATION

Now this is probably a good place to tell you that alcohol is a *sedative*, and to point out the implications of that fact. Alcoholism is a chronic, progressive, incurable disease characterized by loss of control over alcohol and other sedatives. The alcoholic has lost control over not just the drug alcohol - for alcohol is basically nothing more than a widely available, socially acceptable, non prescription and inexpensive tranquilizer or sedative. It's one that you go buy in the liquor store or supermarket rather than a pharmacy. But if you look at it as a drug - if you look at what it does to the brain - it's a sedative. It works by putting brain tissue to sleep just lake a tranquilizer or sleeping pill.

You can probably see that we've got a tricky issue here. Because if the alcoholic has lost control over alcohol, that's not the only drug he's lost control over; he's lost control over *all* other sedative drugs as well. And indeed, one of the really big problems in current treatment, at least among the patients I see, is that the majority (60%) are not only abusing ethyl alcohol. They are also abusing minor tranquilizers and sleeping pills - sedative drugs that, interestingly enough, they usually get by prescription legally from physicians who a.) don't know they're treating alcoholics or b.) don't know how to treat alcoholism and don't recognize alcoholism as a disease that is characterized also by loss of control over the very drugs that they are prescribing.

So you can rapidly end up with someone who is not only addicted to ethyl alcohol but also hooked on tranquilizers and sleeping pills; and he'll probably switch back and forth from one to the other. Or he may stay dry but hooked on pills, in which case the basic disease goes right on destroying him. But the chances are that the alcoholic will mix liquor and pills, and that will only speed the destruction process. Mixing sedatives compounds the risks tremendously. Probably all of us have read in the papers about famous celebrities killed by accidental overdoses of combined sleeping pills, tranquilizers and ethyl alcohol. It's becoming an extremely common cause of death.

All right, we now know what alcoholism is: a chronic, progressive, incurable disease characterized by a loss of control over alcohol and other sedatives. This is the definition I like to use clinically. If I have a patient sitting in my office and I'm trying to make a decision "Does Jack or Jane have alcoholism?" this is the definition I go to work with. Loss of control is the most important clinical factor. Does this individual have a predictable behavior when he drinks? If he does, then he's not alcoholic. But if his behavior isn't predictable when he drinks - if he simply can't tell what will happen next - then I know the disease has got him in hand.

HOW MEDICINE DEFINES DISEASE

But then I'm a physician specializing in the diagnosis and treatment of alcoholism. Many doctors, maybe including your family physician, refuse to this day to believe that alcoholism is a disease: they see it as a character or moral flaw, a simple lack of will power. And we understand why they do. So for them and perhaps for the lingering doubters among you we need to talk about alcoholism in a still more specific and scientific way. We need to do this because it can help rescue some people from alcoholism.

When we doctors talk about a disease, we usually start off by asking about the cause or "etiology". But we're going to put that off for just a minute. Every good story needs a certain amount of suspense.

Though doctors like to talk about a disease's etiology, necessity compels us to look first at *signs and symptoms.* Signs are the physical marks a doctor can literally see in a sick individual: the red welts on the skin we call hives, for example, or the fever that accompanies pneumonia or the sugar that a diabetic will have in his urine. Symptoms are the complaints that bring a sick person to the doctor's office in the first place. A diabetic will tell you that he's tired all the time or insatiably thirsty. Our question here, of course, is: are there unique signs and symptoms for the mysterious disease we call alcoholism?

Absolutely! There are probably more than for most diseases, and we now know a good deal about them. Forty years ago, Dr. E.M. Jellinek in this country and Dr. Max Glatt in England put together a precise description of the progression of alcoholism from early stages to middle and late stages. They had the symptoms down so well that they could see a patient only once and tell what stage of the disease he was in. The stages of a person's disease, incidentally, are what physicians call pathogenesis.

I won't go through all the signs and symptoms - there are 50 or 60 common ones, and many others not so common - but I do want to mention a few that might be called highlights. In the early stages, for instance, you have what is known as relief drinking. An individual uses alcohol to get relief from something: physical pain, emotional pain, money worries - it could be anything. Drunk driving commonly occurs in the early stages of alcoholism. Also memory blackouts. That's a period of amnesia that occurs while the person is drinking. Aunt Jane may look fairly normal - you know she's been drinking, but she's still functioning, she's still walking around the room, carrying on conversations, etc. But tomorrow Jane will be amnesiac; she won't recall what happened the night before. It's a very common symptom of alcoholism, and indeed if you know an individual who's had that experience more than once or twice, the odds are that person is alcoholic. Relief drinking, drunk driving, blackouts - these are all early stage symptoms.

Then we get to the middle stages of the disease. This is commonly called the *crucial stage*, because it's here that most alcoholics can be detected and gotten into treatment. It's also the period when, if you don't get them into treatment, the chances for recovery go way down; so it is in fact extremely crucial.

It is in this stage that we see the classic symptoms: absenteeism from work, poor job performance, financial problems, family problems, the changes in moral and ethical behavior that tend to occur as the disease gets worse and help the alcoholic to be so disliked. These are the signs and symptoms that make the disease fairly visible and detectable - it could be a lucky time if the afflicted person somehow starts to get some treatment. And treatment is certainly needed because this is the beginning of alcoholism's physical problems as well. It's toward the end of this middle or crucial stage that the liver starts to go bad. Marital problems on a physical basis - impotence - begin to show up. The alcoholic is in sadder shape than ever he knows now. The trouble is that he's probably not sober enough to know how much it hurts.

And we're about to cross a gray line here. Once the deterioration of the body starts, the alcoholic has entered the late or chronic stages of the disease.

Most of us, when we think of an alcoholic, picture the chronic-stage person. *The semi-human down there with the body gone rotten, the liver shot, the brain only flickering a little and about to go out.* Generally we picture the skid row bum who-in fact-makes up 3, maybe 4% of the alcoholics in the world today. Most alcoholics aren't fortunate enough to live to reach that stage. Most will die traumatically - on a highway, or at home with a cigarette that they forgot to put out and it burns up their bed with them in it. You probably know how risky it is to spend even one evening drunk in the modern world. It takes 20 to 25 years of heavy drinking to reach the chronic stage. There aren't a lot of veterans.

LIFE-SAVING VALUE OF DISEASE ACCEPTANCE

All right. We've now become very gloomy - which is the natural pathogenesis of alcoholism when it goes its way without treatment. But the wonderful thing about the disease concept is that it allows us to detect the alcoholic's symptoms and get him into treatment before the damage is irreversible. And once in the proper treatment, complete and total recovery is highly probable.

So yes - thank God - there are signs and symptoms of alcoholism. I can take first year medical students and teach them the signs and symptoms in an hour, and then they will be able to make the right diagnosis. But - I'm having to say but a lot in the story - far too few medical students are taught to recognize alcoholism's signs and symptoms. Far too few, even today are taught to recognize alcoholism as a disease. This, I honestly feel, is a national, indeed worldwide disgrace.

In the United States today roughly 34.5 out of every 36 people who have alcoholism are going to die from it, one way or another. It's going to kill them. And they will never have been treated for it. Oh, they will have been treated. They'll have been treated in a lot of hospitals - they'll have been in there for all the physical problems that go with being an alcoholic: the stomach problems, the liver, the pancreas, the nerves. They may even have been frequently hospitalized in psychiatric units where all kinds of psychiatric labels are attached to them. They will be "manic depressives" because they have episodes of depression regularly. Well, I'd be depressed too if my wife had left me, if I'd lost my job and my body was rotting out from underneath me. I think I might have episodes of depression.

Alcoholics get all kinds of labels stuck on them. And a lot of treatment - frequently with other sedative drugs which drives the addiction in even more deeply and shoves the alcoholic downhill even faster. Treatment is available but it's often simply the wrong treatment. Therefore, naturally...the alcoholic dies.

The luckier ones die. About half of one per cent of every 36 - will go insane. They will wind up with physical brain damage: "wet brain", which you've probably heard about. So much of the brain tissue is destroyed in these late stages of alcoholism that the only thing to be done with the alcoholic is to put him in a state hospital or nursing home. There we feed him, clothe him, bathe him and try to keep booze out of his reach. He'll still be smart enough to sneak liquor, if that's in any way possible. But he won't have the brains to take care of anything else.

So a significant number of alcoholics will eventually have their minds destroyed by the disease. About 34 out of 36 will be killed by it in one way or another. One out of 36 will get treatment, will recover and get well. That's a tragic statistic. It's tragic because it's unnecessary. For we do have the proper treatment now - the treatment of alcoholism as a primary disease - and with proper treatment these awful numbers are changed completely around.

Look at these statistics. Let's say that we've caught someone in the throes of middle stage alcoholism. The classic case is someone who is still employed but has been forced into treatment by an employer because of deteriorating job performance. In this situation, recovery rates are as high as 80% : 8 out of 10 middle-stage alcoholics can get well! We can't expect the same for late or chronic-stage alcoholics: but even there-among skid row types, the worst cases you can think of - the recovery rate runs from 25 to 30-35%. By "recovery," I mean people regaining their health and going back to normal, functioning, working lives. This is another strange aspect of the disease we call alcoholism. There are very few chronic, progressive, incurable illnesses where 25 to 80% of those who have them can get well again.

ALCOHOLISM - THE CAUSE

Now we obviously have an interesting mystery here. We've described a certain disease, and we've said that without the proper treatment for it, the chances for recovery are almost nil. We've said that with the proper treatment, the chances for recovery are pretty good. Why on earth, then, aren't most alcoholics getting proper treatment?

Remember when several pages back we started to talk about the "etiology" - the cause - of a disease? What causes alcoholism? Many layman, and unfortunately many helping professionals, would ascribe it to the alcoholics personal weakness, his lack of character and will power, his simple inability to say "No" to a temptation that the rest of us find the gumption to refuse. But we're mainly remembering obnoxious, often disgusting "drunks" when we think this way. Since its beginning in 1935 Alcoholics Anonymous has helped millions of people recover from severe drinking problems. Modern treatment centers have helped many more. How have these millions suddenly developed the will power to *quit* drinking? The weak character theory seems to raise more questions than it answers.

What causes alcoholism? We're not entirely sure, and we should admit that. I can't tell you I know the etiology of alcoholism, because I don't. But we do have more knowledge about what might cause it than we do about most other disease. We certainly shouldn't say as some doctors will that because we don't know the cause of alcoholism, it can't be described as a real disease at all. If that were true, then cancer and diabetes and arteriosclerosis aren't real diseases either; because we don't really know what causes them. Yet every day I hear professionals say that about alcoholism. It's a backdoor way of saying that alcoholism is caused by weak character. Or it might be just the bad luck of the alcoholic. Or maybe a voodoo curse.

THE FAMILY CONNECTION

What causes alcoholism? We don't know for sure, but we now have some pretty good ideas. Medical research has shown, for example, that alcoholism runs in families. You've probably noticed that tendency from your own observation. Family histories taken from patients indicate that, 95% of the time, yes indeed, the mother had a drinking problem, or the father did, or an uncle or brother. Usually, when there is one alcoholic in a family, you'll find many more in the background. Nor is this largely a matter of environment - the atmosphere one learns to drink in as one grows up. That question has pretty well been answered in the past 20 years, and especially in the research done in the 1970's. Heredity studies, done all over the world, clearly show that genetics is far more significant in determining whether or not you'll be an alcoholic than any other single factor examined. Genetics is more significant than any other combination of social or environmental factors examined.

Now I'm not saying a person is born an alcoholic. No, I've never met an alcoholic who didn't drink. But I think it is conclusive that some people are indeed predisposed to alcoholism because of their heredity; and if they ever start drinking they run an unbelievable high risk of developing the disease.

TIQs - BIOCHEMICAL CULPRITS

Of course, in medicine we have a lot of diseases that work that way. Diabetes has a high family predisposition. So, probably, does heart disease. Now, when medical science notices a family predisposition toward a disease, it will look for some abnormality in the body chemistry. What about the body chemistry of alcoholics? In just this past 10 years we think we've found it.

Back in 1972, I was attending a medical conference in San Diego, California. Strolling about the hotel conference center, I happened to glance into a meeting room where several distinguished doctors were huddled around a movie projector watching the antics of drunken rats!

One wretched rodent in particular caught my eye. The animal was so intoxicated that he literally had to squirm and crawl across his cage to reach a saucer containing alcohol and water. Once there, he dropped his snout into the solution up to his eyeballs - and drowned! My gosh! I thought, the poor creature reminds me of some of my patients!

I was fascinated because I knew that the ordinary laboratory rat will not willingly drink alcohol. Place a saucer of water alongside a saucer of ten percent alcohol and water and the rat will sensibly choose the water over the mixed drink every time. And some rats hate alcohol so much that they will die of thirst before touching water with alcohol in it!

How did the research scientists turn a sober, sensible rat into a carousing rat? Further inquiries gave me the answer. Using sophisticated lab techniques, the scientists bathed the rat's brain with a chemical called tetrahydroisoquinolins or, mercifully, TIQ for short. Before proceeding, I must caution the reader that we are about to enter the area of theoretical biochemistry - and controversy. There is a very strong tradition in Western Judeo-Christian culture that we are all born with identical potentials for good and bad behavior.

The devil leads some of us astray while the authorities - ministers, police, parents, teachers - try mightily to keep us on the straight and narrow.

This is the source of shame felt by most people with alcoholism. Strong people of good character can resist temptation, while the weak - willed fall prey to Satan's wiles and deceptions. The idea that the underlying cause of chemical addiction, and its resultant antisocial or asocial behavior, might be inborn, morally neutral, and beyond the reach of sermons, lectures and punishment does not set well with those who believe people choose to be drunks or drug addicts.

Back to biochemistry. A few years before the drunken rat experiments, researchers were able to make TIQs in the test tube using a chemical called acetaldehyde.

Now the addiction sleuths were really on to something! As you read the next few paragraphs, keep that picture in your mind of a rat who detests alcohol so much it will die of thirst before drinking a weak solution of alcohol and water. Put a single injection of TIQs into the rat's brain, offer it alcohol and it will drink nothing else!

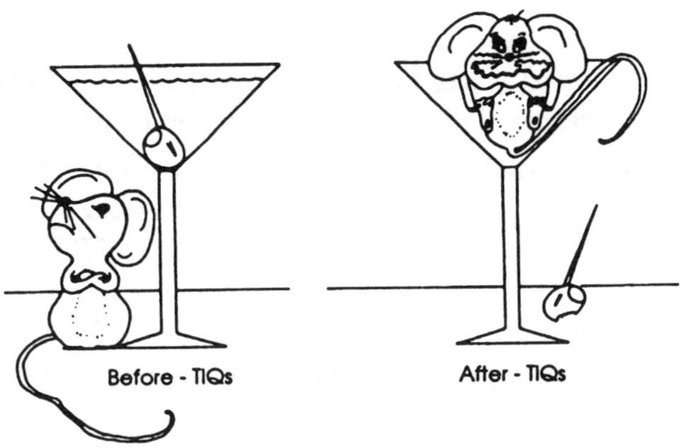

STILL MORE SCIENTIFIC EVIDENCE

Remember, I said we are now in an area of controversial biochemistry. Some critics of the disease model of addiction - the ones who cling to the, in my opinion, ludicrous belief that people choose chemical addiction as a lifestyle, continue to say that science has not conclusively demonstrated the biochemical or genetic cause of addiction. This is quite true. But we know as much or more about what might cause addiction as we do about every other major disease. In the past, I have hesitated to share a lot of the research in these booklets because of its highly technical nature. But I think my patients are intelligent enough to understand that all medical research is intermediate, incremental and tentative. At the beginning of this booklet, I said much news from medical science is bad, that all sorts of environmental factors and food items are now thought to cause this or that disease. But nothing is ever this conclusive or absolute. Most major killers - cancer, heart disease - do not have a single type of cause, but are thought to be brought about by a complex combination of lifestyle, environmental, genetic factors. This is precisely the case with addiction disease. Keep this in mind as you read the following.

RAT ROLE MODELS

As we have seen, addiction researchers have been repeatedly helping rats stagger drunkenly off the straight and narrow. Actually, there is no longer any need to cause a rat to drink itself into alcoholism. We have been able to breed ready made genetic alcoholism in rodents.

Researchers have carefully examined the brains of the rats born genetically alcoholic and have made even more intriguing discoveries. Rats that love alcohol were found to be very deficient in a chemical known as "met-enkephalin". Met-enkephalin is one of the chemicals in our brains known as the endorphins. The endorphins are our brains own natural opiates. When we are stressed or in pain the endorphins are released from our brain cells and help us cope with stress and pain. A deficiency of endorphins has also been shown to create a state of pleasurelessness and depression. In short the alcohol preferring rats are born without enough of mother nature's own feel good chemical, the endorphins. (Not surprisingly, when the brains of alcohol hating rats were examined they were found to have an adequate supply of met-enkephalin.)

Now what does this have to do with TIQs? Well further research has shown that the presence of TIQs in the brains of the alcohol hating rats will cause the production of endorphins to be shut off. It seems the brain mistakes the TIQs for endorphins and shuts down production of endorphins. It is not hard to hypothesize that when the endorphin levels fall low enough and one stops drinking and making TIQs that there will then be a state of pleasurelessness and depression caused by the absence of adequate endorphins. The quick answer to this depression is familiar to every alcoholic - drink and make more TIQs to take the place of the natural endorphins. The disease and its terrible consequences thus progress.

Other research has added to our knowledge of the neurochemistry of alcoholism. In studying early onset alcoholic males, it was discovered that they had an abnormal EEG (electrical brain wave study). This abnormal wave was referred to as the P3 or P300 wave. The question: was this abnormal brain wave a consequence of the years of alcoholic drinking these men have been through or could it be a marker of their illness? This question was resolved when the researchers studied the brain waves of the sons of early onset alcoholics who had not yet started drinking or drugging and discovered the same abnormal P3 wave. This EEG finding appears to be a genetic marker for early onset alcoholism.

Just recently it has been discovered that early onset alcoholics also appear to have a deficiency of an enzyme called MAO (mono-amine-oxidase) in a blood cell known as the platelet. We know that the level of MAO in the platelet is a reflection of the amount of MAO in the brain. In the brain MAO is an important enzyme that is involved in the regulation of critical brain chemicals such as seritonin, norepinephrine, and dopamine. These are exactly the same chemicals that have been found to be affected by drugs such as cocaine and amphetamine and that have been implicated in the development of significant depression. Still more evidence of the role of neurochemistry in the development not only of alcoholism but of all drug addiction.

GOING BACK TO SOME BASICS

But again, one of the key research findings is what apparently happens to the chemical acetaldehyde in the brains of alcoholic rats - and people. As you read the following keep in mind that TIQs will instantly turn an alcohol - hating rat into a rat with full blown alcoholism.

When the normal adult drinker takes in alcohol, it is very rapidly eliminated at the rate of about one drink per hour. The body first converts the alcohol into the previously mentioned acetaldehyde. This is very toxic stuff, and if it were to build up inside us, we would get violently sick; and indeed we could die. But mother nature helps us to get rid of acetaldehyde very quickly. She efficiently changes it into acetic acid, which we know as vinegar, and then changes it a couple of more times - into carbon dioxide and water - which is happily eliminated through our kidneys and lungs. That's what happens to normal drinkers. It also happens with alcoholic drinkers, but they get something more.

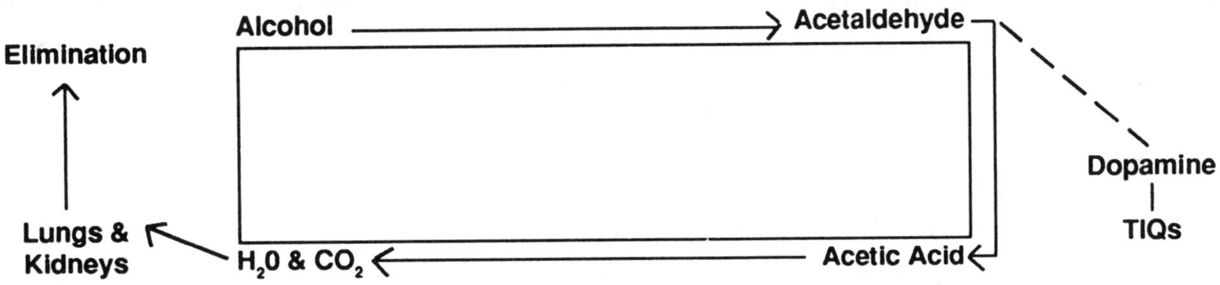

There is growing evidence that something additional happens in the alcoholic. In them, a very small amount of poisonous acetaldehyde is not eliminated; instead it goes to the brain where, through a very complicated biochemical process, it winds up as this TIQs I mentioned before. Researchers have found out fascinating things about TIQs. Let me tell you a little about them here.

First, TIQ is manufactured right in the brain, and **it only occurs in the brain of the alcoholic drinker; it doesn't happen in the brain of the normal social drinker of alcohol.**

Second, TIQs have been found to be highly addictive. It was tried in experimental use with animals during the Second World War, when we were looking for a pain killer less addicting than morphine. TIQs were a pretty good pain killer, all right, but it couldn't be used on humans. **It turned out to be much more addicting than morphine.** So scientists had to forget about it, and they've left it all these years up on some dusty shelf.

THE PIECES BEGIN TO FIT

You see how beautifully these laboratory findings fit in with what we specialists in alcoholism have long noticed in our clinics. Uncle Jack is brought in, and he's drunk again, and even though it's slowly killing him, he somehow can't stop drinking. When he is sober enough we will get a family history. Yes, there are other alcoholics in his family; there is a family predisposition - an abnormality in the family body chemistry - which we only saw the shadow of before. But now we see it much more clearly: it's a predisposition toward making TIQs.

Now alcoholics don't intend to make TIQs when they start drinking. They don't mean for their brains to manufacture something stronger than morphine - they've been warned about the evils of narcotics all their lives. But they've heard a good deal less about the evils of alcoholism. Most normal Americans take a drink now and then, and the young alcoholics-to-be want to be normal. So they take a drink now and then, too.

Unfortunately, the alcoholics-to-be aren't normal. That's too bad for them but then it could have been a lot worse: they could have been born blind or with crippled arms or legs. On the other hand, of course, potential alcoholics certainly would know about the blindness or the crippling disability. But they don't know about the predisposition toward TIQ - making their brain chemistry has inherited. Nobody knew about it until fairly recently. So Jack and Jane and a new generation of alcoholics have their first drinks, and everything seems cool.

The alcoholic has his or her early drinks, and now we can go back to our little lesson in biochemistry. The alcoholic's body, like yours and mine, changes the alcohol into acetaldehyde, and then it changes most of that into carbon dioxide and water, which in the end it kicks out through the kidneys and lungs. Except, of course, that alcoholic's bodies won't kick all these chemicals out. The alcoholics brain likes them for some reason, and holds a few bits back and transforms them into TIQs.

So the alcoholic-to-be starts drinking, and he or she may well be very moderate at first. Just a few on Saturday nights. Maybe a couple of beers with football games on TV. Maybe a nip or two to calm down while fixing dinner for the family. Two or three drinks to quiet the jitters before high school graduation. In the beginning, the alcoholic-to-be only gets seriously drunk, say, once or twice a year. So far, so good. But all this time the alcoholic brain is humming away in there building its little cache of TIQs. At some point, maybe sooner, maybe later, the alcoholic will cross over a shadowy line into a whole new way of life.

Now medical science still doesn't know where this line is - doesn't know how much TIQs an individual brain will pile up before the big event happens. Some predisposed people cross the line while they are teenagers - or earlier! It won't occur in others until they are 30 or 40 or maybe even retired. But once it does happen, the alcoholic will be as hooked on alcohol as he would have been hooked on heroin if he had been shooting that instead - and for very similar chemical reasons! Now comes the *loss of control* we talked about earlier in the story. Now its chronic, progressive, incurable nature is obvious to practically everyone who knows the alcoholic. Now it is all too clearly a disease. And now - all too often - it's a disease that will mainly get treated with other *sedatives*. Far too often alcohol addiction is treated with pills that keep the disease raging. When we're done, if the alcoholic is still alive, he'll be about as functional as the TIQed rat.

GOOD NEWS

But then I did promise you good news, didn't I? Well, we're just about to it, and you may well understand it already. Alcoholism is a disease - and that's the good news. Alcoholism is not the alcoholic's fault - and that's good news, too. Alcoholics can today get proper treatment for the disease, which is certainly good news, and that treatment begins when we tell them these facts. The alcoholic patients I see are usually hugely relieved to hear that it's not their fault, because they've been carrying tons of guilt along with the alcoholism - and that guilt was often worse than useless.

Now instead of guilt, the alcoholic person can take on some responsibility. Now that the alcoholic knows the facts, he or she can, with treatment, take the responsibility of stopping the drinking; alcoholics can refuse to put more TIQs in their brains and they can refuse to reactivate the TIQs that are already there.

WHAT NOW ?

For most of human history alcoholism was considered a hopeless condition. Not so today, in fact it is the only chronic, incurable and ultimately fatal if arrested disease from which a majority of victims can expect 100% recovery. But, sadly, as with other chronic illnesses, relapse is common. *And each relapse statistically increases the odds against full recovery.* This is why treatment professionals and AA insist on complete and continuous abstinence. There has been some talk lately of teaching chronic, relapse - prone alcoholics to have shorter, lower consequence drinking bouts, or relapses. This in my opinion is madness and medically irresponsible. The idea has about as much validity as trying to teach alcoholics to have a single glass of wine with dinner. We must work to avoid relapse for the same reasons we work to keep cancer in remission or keep people with heart disease from having heart attacks. *We never know if the next attack , tumor or relapse will be fatal!*

RELAPSE PREVENTION

Relapse prevention is a big issue today. Entire, inpatient treatment programs are devoted to the subject. I ordinarily would not try to treat people in the pages of a booklet. But I would like to offer a few suggestions based on more than 20 years of treating addiction disease.

THE BIOCHEMISTRY OF RECOVERY

Many of my patients want to become happy, joyous, free, physically fit, financially successful, and an inspirational AA role model overnight. Years of being mired in a debilitating disease has made them impatient for the good life once they believe they can recover. But it takes time to physically and mentally recover from any serious illness and addiction is no exception. First of all, the brain has more or less physically damaged. The regular impact of alcohol and drugs has thrown many of the brain's delicate neurochemicals out of whack. Time will restore these systems to what is normal for each individual. Plus there has been a regular interference into ordinary, sober, psychological, and emotional operations. If a person has spent years deadening or enhancing feelings with a chemical, the brain has stopped learning how to deal with stress any other way. Emotional skills, like physical skills, must be refined through repetition and practice.

All this makes recovery tricky and relapse much more common than it needs to be.

Remember...

1. It will take a few months for physical healing, longer to develop emotional coping skills for the ordinary stress of daily living. Don't be impatient. Find support and take it one day at a time.

2. Relapse is never trivial. It's like a person with heart disease having a heart attack. The next one might be fatal!

3. If you remain clean and sober, there will come a time when you will be much happier than at any time during your active addiction.

PLEASURE / PURPOSE PRINCIPLE

I want to share something I have been telling my patients for many years. There is a tendency among recovering people toward self-flagellation and somber penitence. People used to go off to nunneries and monasteries after too much high living.

Certainly, it is good to make amends to people you have hurt by your behavior while under the influence. But whatever you might have done while in the grip of addiction disease, does not mean you have forfeited your right to enjoy life. In fact, if you don't learn to enjoy yourself, your chances of recovery are not good. I'm not a philosopher or guru, but it seems to me that general happiness involves two things; pleasure and purpose.

PLEASURE

Pain has important, but limited survival value. Pleasure and memories of pleasure drive us to eat, have sex, pay attention to our children and mates, and keep our spirits up when times are bad. We might say pleasure is the root of hope and optimism. This is why I tell my patients to enjoy themselves. Have fun! Play!

PLAY, BUT BE CAREFUL

The most dangerous thing of all for recovering addicts is something called "euphoric memory". There was at least one time in a users life when the drug alcohol did everything it was supposed to do - and more. After all, that's why you kept using it! Most people think "euphoric memory" is simply a memory of feeling real good in itself. This is not true. Euphoric memory has many details: place, setting, drugs, bottles, cans - a rock concert, a party, a bar, and so on. In short, euphoric memory can be any combination of times when you were drinking or using and felt terrific, and all the elements present at the time. Cocaine addicts talk about instant craving at the mere sight of the drug or drug paraphernalia. Alcoholics tell of becoming uncomfortable around certain holidays, or passing down the street of a favorite bar. You see, human beings remember pleasure much better than we remember pain. If this were not so, we'd have come to a paralyzed, phobic evolutionary dead end a long time ago.

PURPOSE

It helps to have a reason for living beyond the enjoyment of daily pleasures. I don't mean "purpose" in some grandiose sense - ending world hunger or establishing peace on earth - but realistic, obtainable personal life goals and objectives. Sort out your dreams and find a purposeful reality. Dreams and fantasies are definitely not silly or childish. Many accomplished people will tell you (if they're honest) that they visualized their success, even at times when the possibility of achieving it seemed remote. In fact, strong daydreams of success are about the only thing I know of that will sustain us though disappointments and setbacks.

Here's how to turn daydreams into achievable purpose. All achievements and success involve a series of steps. For example I have accomplished my goal of being a physician. But I first finished high school, pre-med, medical school, internship, etc. And all this was built on even smaller steps; passing exams, getting to class on time, etc. Break your dreams down into doable, daily steps. Decide what you want to do in life, and list the steps necessary to do it. Work on the steps one at a time. Again, any dream or purpose is fine. Becoming a mother or father or golf player can be just as engaging as becoming the next U.S. congressman from your district.

DISEASE CONCEPT OVERVIEW

I. American Medical Association Definition = Alcoholism is an illness characterized by preoccupation with alcohol; by loss of control over its consumption, such as to usually lead to intoxication or drinking done by chronicity; by progression and the tendency to relapse. It is typically associated with physical disability and impaired emotion, occupational, and/or social adjustments as a direct consequence of persistent and effective use.

Dr. David Ohlms' Definition = Alcoholism is a chronic, progressive, incurable disease characterized by loss of control over alcohol and other sedatives.

Chronic = Lasts a long time.

Progressive = Alcoholism doesn't go away, it gets worse after long periods of sobriety, and can be reactivated by a single drink.

Incurable = We can't return to normal drinking. We can return to a normal life, but only if we stop drinking.

Loss of control = Once the alcoholic takes that first drink after a period of being sober or abstinent, he can't predict with any reliability whether he's going to have a normal or abnormal drinking episode. Therefore, we don't control alcohol, it controls us.

This is the major factor in defining alcoholism - can we predict our behavior every time we drink?

Alcohol is a sedative drug. We've lost control over the use of other sedative drugs, i.e., tranquilizers and sleeping pills.

II. There are signs and symptoms for every disease. Dr. E.M. Jellinek and Dr. Max Glatt describe alcoholism in three clearly definable stages; early, middle, and late.

Early Stage Symptoms are:

Relief Drinking - To get relief from physical or emotional pain, worries, etc.

Blackouts - Any period of amnesia which occurs while drinking. More than two episodes are indicative of alcoholism.

Drunk driving - Driving while intoxicated, no matter how slight, shows impaired thinking.

Middle Stage Symptoms - This is the crucial stage for getting treatment. Classic symptoms: Absenteeism, poor job performance, financial problems, family problems, changes in normal or ethical behavior.

Late or Chronic Stage Symptoms - End stages of body deterioration. Only one in three alcoholics will recover.

III. The cause or etiology of alcoholism.

Most research shows that alcoholism is genetic. See handout on genetics. Ninety-five percent of alcoholics have alcoholism in their family. **Genetics is the single most important factor in determining whether you will be an alcoholic or not.**

A. Production of TIQ's
A faulty gene responsible for the proper breakdown, or metabolism of alcohol is probably what is being passed on genetically generation to generation.

In a normal person, alcohol is broken down like this:

Normal Alcohol Metabolism

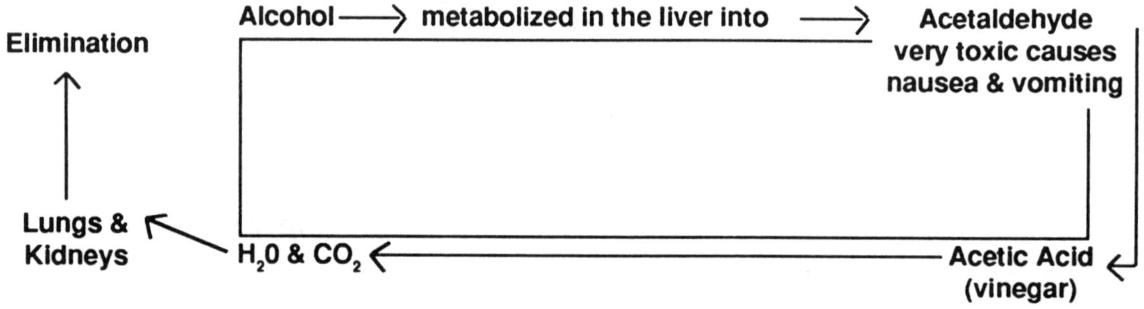

In the alcoholic, not all of the acetaldehyde is removed. Part of it goes through a series of chemical reactions in the brain and makes TIQ's.

Alcoholic Alcohol Metabolism

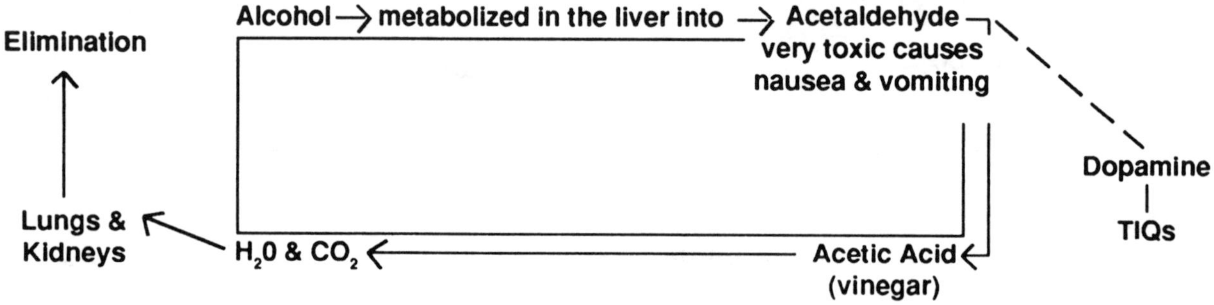

TIQ is a morphine-type substance found only in the brains of alcoholics.
This is important to understand for two reasons:

1. When the brain makes TIQ's, a morphine type chemical, **it stops making its own morphine type chemical** , the endorphins, which are responsible for helping us deal with pain. Endorphins make us "feel good." So when we quit drinking, we have a lower level of endorphins in our brains and feel somewhat depressed or "flat". We start drinking again to make more TIQs and feel normal.

2. **TIQs are highly addicting** - more addicting than morphine. Like any other addict addicted to morphine or heroin, we need to keep drinking alcohol to keep making the TIQ's our brain has made and become addicted to. This helps explain loss of control.

3. **TIQ's don't go away.** Once in the brain, they stay there. This explains how after long periods of abstinence, an alcoholic who drinks starts up where he left off. It's as if he never stopped. This explains the progression of the disease.

   A. Type II alcoholics appear to have an abnormal P3 wave.

   B. Type II alcoholics also appear to have MAO deficiencies. The MAO enzyme is involved with regulating other brain neurotransmitters like serotonin, norepinephrine, and dopamine.

IV. Recovery

While we are not responsible for our genetics, once we understand the facts about our disease, we are totally responsible for our recovery. One-hundred percent of alcoholics can recover. Alcoholics can refuse to put more TIQ's into their brains and they can refuse to reactivate the TIQ's which are already there.

Each relapse statistically increases the odds against full recovery. This is why recovery means complete and total abstinence. Due to our brain chemistry causing loss of control, we never know when our next drink or drug will be fatal.

It takes time to recover physically and mentally.
Give it time.
Use supports.
Avoid triggering "euphoric memory."
Have fun!

DISEASE CONCEPT LECTURE FOLLOW-UP

It is important to have the client's *"identify-in"* immediately following the Disease Concept Lecture. The lecture opens them up to the concept of being chemically dependent, this follow-up helps them *"claim"* the initial aspects discussed in the lecture.

Instructions: Following the lecture, pass around the accompanying handouts. Provide ten to twenty minutes to complete. Have each group member read their answers aloud in group. The group responds by giving feedback to that person relating to whether they agree or disagree with their responses.

Note: This is intended to be a simple introduction to being chemically dependent. Obviously, the facilitator can make the group more "in depth," but it's a good introductory tool for reinforcing the client's willingness to start to accept their chemical dependence. Reinforcing their positive behavior will:

1. Help decrease the initial shame about being chemically dependent so that later they can be more specific about their use.

2. Show the client that they are capable of doing *"the work"*.

3. Keep them motivated and hooked into their peers.

This group can also begin to identify some areas of denial. Again, at this initial level of treatment, it is important to keep it light, as heavy confrontation in the initial stage of treatment only causes a defensive response and lack of trust.

An example of feedback - *"It looks like you can see and accept that your disease has been chronic and progressive, and that you have tolerance. I don't hear that you see much loss of control or significant consequences. What does the rest of the group see?......This is a very good start."* Then leave it at that. Even if their work is awful or completely dishonest, leave the client with some ego strength. This is done by positively reframing something they may not have specifically wanted to say. For example, *"You **really** see how long you've been drinking. Good for you."* Period.

HANDOUT # 3

DISEASE CONCEPT

The Disease Concept Lecture stresses that chemical dependency is:
Chronic = Lasts a long time.
Progressive = It gets worse.
Incurable = We can't return to normal drinking.

It is manifested by:
Loss of Control = Can't predict when we can stop with one or two drinks.
Tolerance = The ability to use more and more of the chemical, exceeding "recommended doses."
Consequences = Despite problems directly related to using/drinking, we continue to use.

This is an introduction to your Step 1 work.
Give an example for each of the above.

Keep it simple:

1. **My disease is chronic:** Describe how long you have had it. Example: *"I drank from 11-years old until 45- years old, a total of 34 years."*

2. **My disease is progressive:** Give example of how it has become worse. Example: *"When I was 16-years old, I only drank on weekends. Now I drink daily."*

3. **My disease is incurable:** Give an example of not being able to return to normal use.

4. **Loss of control**: Give an example of loss of control.

5. **Tolerance**: Give an example of change in tolerance.

6. **The biggest consequence has been:**

MORE ON THE CAUSES OF ALCOHOLISM

Research shows that both genetic and environmental factors contribute to alcoholism.

GENETICS: There is probably a combination of genes, not a single gene responsible for causing alcoholism. Genes are organized and stored in structures called chromosomes which are located in the nucleus of the cell. Essentially they carry the blueprint for the body to synthesize proteins. If the gene is defective, the resulting protein manufactured is defective or abnormal and will function abnormally.

Researchers are exploring traits which may be linked to alcoholism susceptibility in three areas:

1. Behavioral traits - Violent and impulsive behavior is more apparent in Type II alcoholism.

2. Physiological traits - Abnormal EEG's. Early studies showed the reduction of P3 brain waves in Type II (high risk) alcoholics, who had become abstinent. The male children of Type II alcoholics showed the same reduction in the P3 wave. Smaller P3 brain waves may be a marker for alcoholism susceptibility in these children. It is still unclear how women are affected genetically.

3. Biochemical traits - At present, researchers are extensively studying two biochemical markers for genetic involvement with alcoholism.

   A. MAO (Monoamine oxidase). MAO is an enzyme which is involved in the metabolism (or manufacturing) of several neurotransmitters (brain chemicals) which are involved with alcoholism. In the highly genetic Type II alcoholism, abnormally low levels of MAO are found in the blood platelets of alcoholics and their not yet drinking sons. It may be possible in the near future to determine the predisposition to alcoholism by drawing the blood MAO levels in children of alcoholic males.

   B. AC (adenosine cyclase). AC is found in the central nervous system (brain tissues) and is involved with the formation of chemicals responsible for some behavioral responses. The production of these enzymes is lower in alcoholics.

Animal studies - There have been lots of animal studies done on selectively bred or genetically altered animals. One of the more significant studies was done on genetically bred rats. Two types of rats were studies and compared:

P rats = alcohol preferring rats
NP rats = alcohol non-preferring rats

The alcohol preferring P rats were born with lower levels of the brain **neurotransmitters serotonin and dopamine.** These are brain chemicals which allow us to feel pleasure. *The rats actually choose alcohol over water to drink.* This is because by **ingesting alcohol,** the rats are releasing more of these pleasure stimulating chemicals in their brains, *which they are otherwise lacking*. In addition, these rats were found to perform better after ingesting lower levels of alcohol.

In contrast, the NP rats became sedated with low levels of alcohol and chose not to drink any alcohol. The NP rats could be encouraged to drink alcohol by giving them a reward for drinking (i.e., food). However, these NP rats were never able to reach the same tolerance or alcohol concentrations of the P rats.

This difference in dopamine and serotonin levels also probably accounts for cross addiction. Dopamine is the main chemical involved with cocaine and amphetamine use. Amphetamine type drugs cause an increased release of dopamine in the brain, causing the quick high or euphoric feeling. Once it is released by the brain, the dopamine is quickly used up or re-absorbed back into the brain, which lowers the brain's normal dopamine level. This requires more cocaine or stimulant drug to release more dopamine.

Eventually, the brain's supply is used up. If cocaine is not available, alcohol is used to try to produce the same effect (as seen in rat studies). All of this leads to increased use of the chemical (tolerance) to get the same effect.

Once the pleasure experiencing dopamine is used up in the brain, the individual experiences depression. Simply because the chemicals to feel "good" are gone. This leads to repeated use of the amphetamine.

Other Studies Involving Genetics:

Generation Studies: The factors related to this are not clear, i.e., is it genetic or environmental?

The onset of alcoholism is occuring at a much younger age. A study done in 1984 shows that of the male alcoholic children of male alcoholics, 52 percent were alcohol dependent by age 20. Only 22 percent developed alcoholism between the ages of 26 to 44 years, and less than 10 percent by ages 45 or older. This seems to suggest that the more alcoholism there is in our family tree, the more concentrated it becomes in younger generations.

Racial Studies: There is a large diversity of genetic backgrounds among American racial minorities. The bulk of alcohol research has only begun to examine alcohol trends among minorities since about 1984. While genetics vary greatly even within racial groups, there seem to be some trends. These trends are derived from epidemiological surveys done in 1984, 1986, and 1989.

These studies relate to alcohol only. There is no conclusive research on other substances.

Black Americans:

1. Black and white American men had similar drinking patterns. However, black men had higher abstention rates (29 versus 23 percent) and white men were more likely to be heavier drinkers.

2. Drinking patterns among black and white women were also similar, however, nearly half of black women were more likely to abstain from alcohol (46 versus 34 percent). Of the black women who drank, they tended to be heavier drinkers than their white counterparts. Generally, black men and women show higher rates of abstention and lower rates of drinking than white men and women.

Some important trends showed up in age-related categories:

1. White men drink the heaviest between the ages of 18 and 29 and drink less after that. This is also the same with white women. Both groups are at highest risk for alcohol related problems during these ages.

2. Black men have the highest abstention rates between the ages of 18 through 29, with sharp increases in heavy drinking past age 30. This probably accounts for the much higher incidence of alcohol related health problems of black men, who

have a much higher incidence of cirrhosis and alcohol related cancers. This study did not include social or economical factors, so it is still unclear how the genetics intertwine with the complications resulting from racial discrimination, social, and economic problems.

Hispanics:

1. A sample survey of a cross section of Hispanics (Mexican, Latin American, Cuban, and Puerto Ricans) shows that the prevalence of alcohol related problems is higher among Hispanic men than white or black men, and highest among Mexican-American men.

2. Hispanic women have the highest rate of abstention, drinking once a month or not at all. However, second generation Hispanic women drinking rates parallel those of white women.

3. Male drinking rates increase sharply in their 30's, but drop sharply again by ages 50 through 60. The rate is close to zero for Hispanic women over 60.

Asian-Americans:

1. Asian-Americans are more likely to be abstainers than any other racial group.

2. Japanese men and women have higher drinking rates than other Asian ethnic groups but have very few alcohol related problems, although this is beginning to increase.

3. Asian women have the lowest incidence of drinking of any racial or gender group.

Native Americans & Alaskans:

It is not possible to make generalizations about drinking patterns among tribal groups as there is such a diversity among drinking practices. Some tribes are abstinent while others have high levels of abuse. The extent of alcohol related abuse shows up in the mortality rates which are alcohol caused or related:

1. In 1985, the mortality rate of Native Americans for cirrhosis and chronic liver disease was 29.2 deaths per 100,000 (three times the U.S. death rate of 9.2 per 100,000).

2. Alcoholism death rates are twice as high for men as for women.

3. There are 96.8 deaths per 100,000 between the ages of 45 through 56.

4. While the women drink less, they account for half of the cirrhosis related deaths, indicating higher vulnerability to alcohol in women.

5. Binge drinking is characteristic of many Indian tribal groups, which may be related to higher rates of accidental deaths, homicides, and suicides than the general population.

Referral Source: Alcohol And Health, U.S. Department of Health and Human Services, 1992.

Note to Clinicians:

The National Institute on Alcohol Abuse and Alcoholism has excellent resource materials. The materials are free. We suggest making these materials available to clients by scattering them around your practice setting. Two particularly useful books are "Alcohol Research" and "Alcohol Health". For more detailed research, ask for the "Initial Sensitivity To Alcohol" manual.

To order, call or write:

NACADI 1-800-729-6686

U.S. Department Of Health And Human Services
Public Health Service
Alcohol, Drug Abuse, And Mental Health Administration
National Institute On Alcohol Abuse And Alcoholism
5600 Fishers Lane
Rockville, MD, 20857

GENETICS OF ALCOHOLISM: FAMILY TREE

Introduction:

It is imperative that the client understand that there is overwhelming evidence showing a genetic link between their chemical dependency and their genetic family history. By doing their family tree, the chemically dependent person can begin to step out of their shame about "being the sickest and most disgusting person in my family and on the planet, the one in treatment", by realizing, *"Of course I'm an alcoholic, look at my genetics, I'm **supposed** to be alcoholic."*

The family tree helps to remove some of the shame of being alcoholic by having them see and concretize the concept that

"With these genetics, who wouldn't be alcoholic?"

This can be reframed with them to dissolve some of their shame by introducing a concept of recovery - gratitude. *"Thank God I'm getting treatment when I am. I should be dead from this."*

Goal:

1. **Reinforce the genetic evidence** of the Disease Concept by identifying the genetic family traits they inherited.

2. **Reinforce the Step 1 initial concepts of powerlessness.** For example: *"I am powerless over **being alcoholic**. I can no more change the genetics I inherited in the way I handle alcohol (chemicals) than I can change my genetics with allergies, skin color or body type, which I also inherited."*

3. **Decrease shame** about their family secrets by allowing others to freely explore the secrets with them.

4. **Begin discussions** of alcoholism prevention and intervention with their children who may have the same genetics.

Materials: Family Tree Outline, Colored Pencils

Group Format:
Present the group as discussed in the introduction. Allow a minimum of 30 minutes for the homework or schedule the homework and follow-up within 24 hours.

Group Follow-up:
Have each member present their genetic "case history" to the group explaining their family tree. Let the group provide feedback. Guide their responses to conclude with the idea, *"No wonder you're alcoholic!"* Ask the group if you can hang up their family trees for 24 hours so people can go back to examine them . Let them air their dirty laundry for a while.

Areas Of Resistance:
Most chemically dependent people can be shown to be genetically linked to other alcoholics. While there is some evidence that there may be no alcoholism in a particular family tree, this is **extremely rare** (explain this in the group introduction).

Problem: *"I'm adopted."* or *"There are absolutely no alcoholics in my family at all. I'm it!"*

Responses:

1. *"Possible but highly unlikely. What would happen to your family if you discovered that out of your family of saints, there was an alcoholic human being thrown in the bunch?"*
2. *"Why not?"*
3. *"Here's a dime. Call your* **(mother, brother, cousin)** *and ask them what they remember. Somebody protected you from the secrets. "*
4. *"If you had to guess, which one member in three generations may have drank too much?"*

Rule of thumb: In most dysfunctional families, one family member is the "secret keeper" and knows "stuff" the others don't. Have them identify and contact that member for more information.

HANDOUT # 4

FAMILY TREE SAMPLE

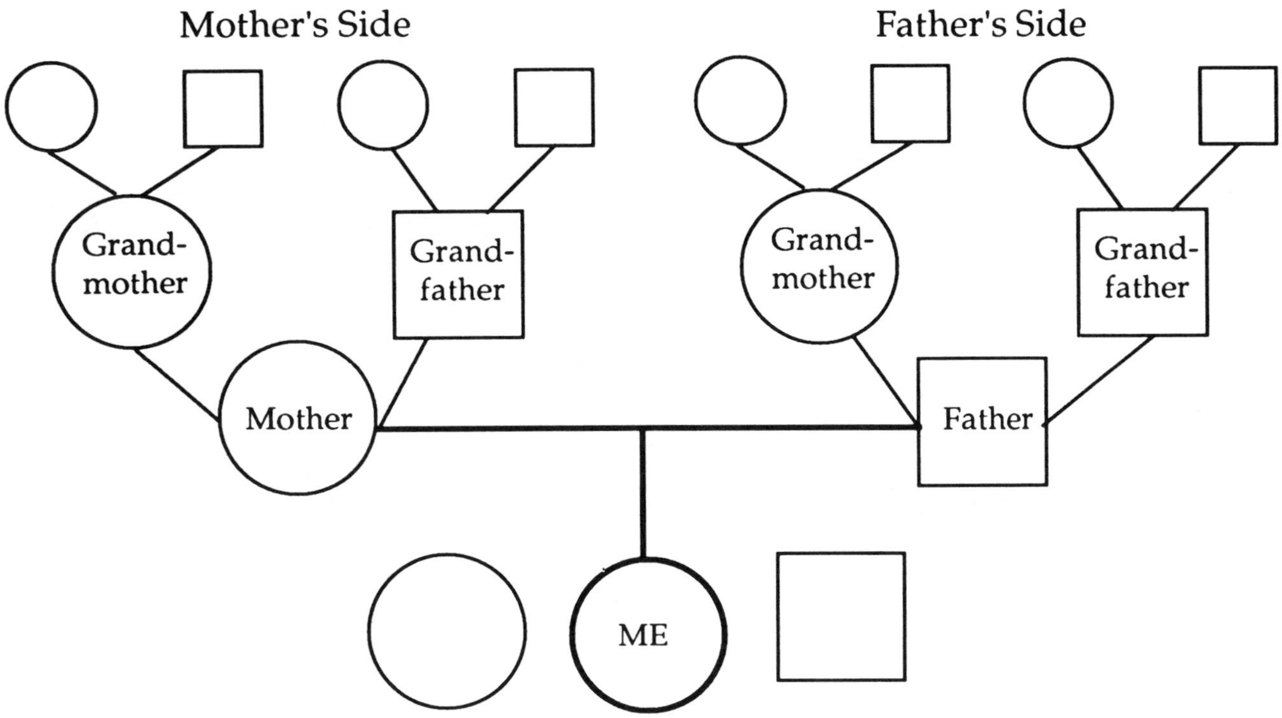

Non genetic variations to add to family tree:
add sexual abuse
physical abuse
divorce
legal problems

Key: = Female = Male

A	=	Alcohol only	C =	Chronic	X	=	Deceased
AD	=	Alcohol & Drugs	B =	Binge use			
D	=	Drugs only					

Other Addictions:

N = Nicotine
ED = Eating disorder (compulsive overeating, bulimia, anorexia)
G = Gambling
MI = Mental Illness
(Describe, i.e., depression, schizophrenia, antisocial, hypochondria, etc.)
V = Violent behavior

HANDOUT # 5

DRAW YOUR FAMILY TREE

MEDICAL ASPECTS OF ALCOHOLISM:

LECTURE INTRODUCTION

This group is best presented as a lecture with discussion. It's a good way to provide information and clear up questions your clients may have about their physical status. Depending upon your type of facility, the group warm-up can be done in any number of ways.

Group Warm-Ups:

If you are a hospital: Hand out copies of the patients' laboratory work, highlighting any abnormalities. Ask them if they know what the results mean, how it affects them. *This is a good time to gather information and assess where the group is with their medical understanding of chemical dependency.*

If you are a non-hospital setting: Warm up the group by doing some simple sociograms. Example of a sociogram:

A. People who know they **have** liver disease, stand over here.
B. People who know they **don't have** liver disease, stand over here.
C. People who **don't know**, stand over here.

Have each person make a statement related to their position.
Example A would say: *"My doctor told me three years ago that I had liver disease."*

Continue the format using different statements, i.e.

People with:	Pancreatitis
	Stomach problems
	Who have thrown up
	Who had withdrawal symptoms
	Who have had more colds this year
	Memory problems
	Accidents, etc.

Then introduce the group.

A good way to explain the presentation is to state that "*Alcohol and most other drugs cross into every tissue of the body, therefore, every organ and organ system is affected. The easiest way to discuss the effect of alcohol is to describe the body systems as the drink is ingested."* It makes it easier for clients to grasp the medical aspects within the framework of *"Picture taking a drink. We'll discuss the medical complications as we follow the drink through the body."*

Choose a group member to be the artist.

Usually a chalkboard is used.

Have the artist draw an outline of a person on the board. Label the organ systems. Ask the group to describe the path alcohol takes in the body to the artist, who will draw and label the body parts in sequence. (It should look something like the following picture.)

Have the artist draw and label these as the group describes it to him.

"Alcohol affects every organ it passes through. It first goes through the ***mouth****, down the* ***esophagus****, into the* ***stomach*** *and into the* ***intestines****, where it's absorbed into the* ***blood****, which takes it to the* ***liver*** *and* ***pancreas****, where it is metabolized, goes into the* ***cardiovascular system****, where it's circulated to the* ***brain and neurological system, bone marrow, reproduction system*** *and through the* ***kidneys****."*

This is the general idea:

Alcohol affects every organ it passes through.

1. It first goes through the mouth,
2. Down the esophagus,
3. Into the stomach,
4. Into the intestines,
5. Into the liver & pancreas,
6. Into the cardiovascular system,
7. Where it's circulated to the brain & neurological system
8. Bone marrow,
9. Reproductive system
10. and excreted by the kidneys.

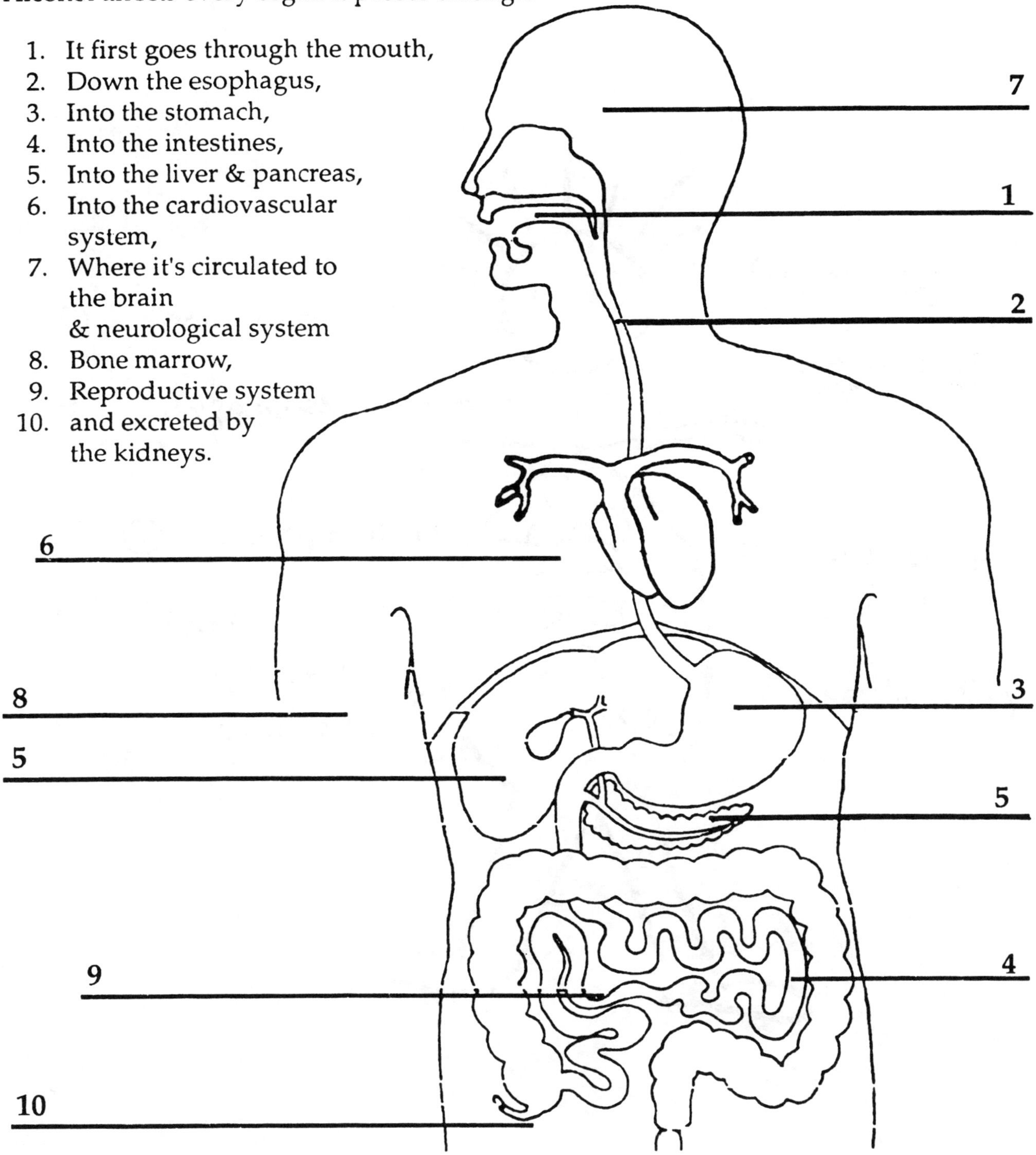

Or, if you draw like us, it could look like this:

THIS WILL ALSO WORK!

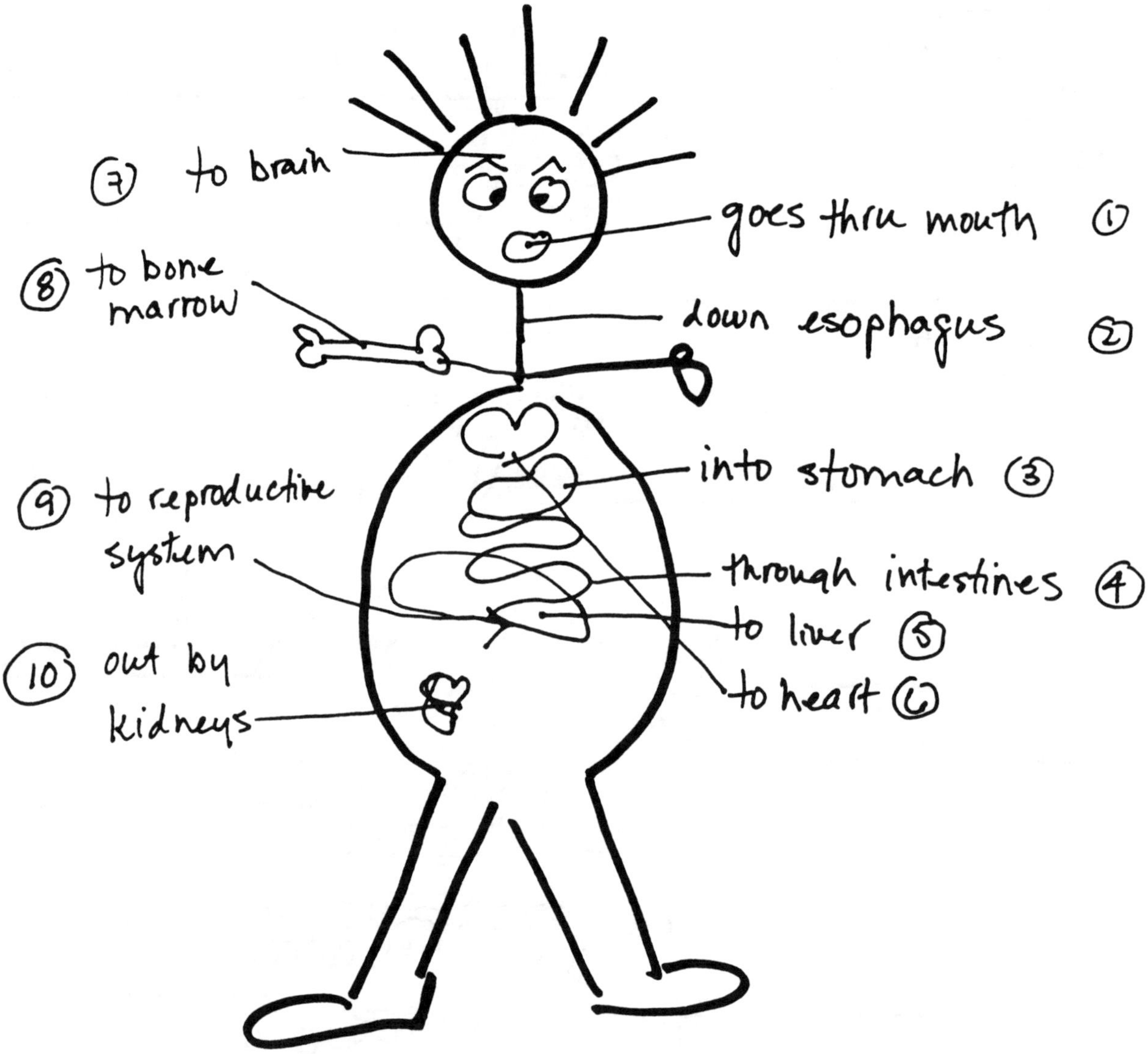

MEDICAL ASPECTS OF ALCOHOLISM: THE LECTURE

Alcohol affects almost every organ system in the body directly or indirectly. Some people may be more vulnerable than others to the medical effects of alcohol for **genetic** reasons. There also seems to be a relationship between medical consequences and the **amount, duration,** and **pattern** (daily vs. binge) of drinking.

While most people are aware of problems like cirrhosis and "wet brain", there are other organ areas affected which are also catastrophic. To examine how alcohol affects the body, it is easiest to envision taking a drink, and follow the affects of alcohol on the organs as it moves through the body.

Alcohol enters the body through the mouth, passes through the esophagus, and enters the stomach and intestines.

General Effects On The Gastrointestinal (GI) Tract

Alcohol affects the stomach and intestines.

The Stomach

The stomach contains many enzymes including the gastric ADH enzyme (alcohol dehydrogenase). In normal drinking, ADH **prevents** alcohol from being directly absorbed from the stomach into the blood system. This is good as the body doesn't want pure alcohol pouring into the blood stream and going directly to the brain where it will damage brain tissue.

Chronic use of alcohol causes damage to the normal stomach lining (or mucosa). This causes three main problems:

1. Breakdown of the normal stomach lining creating gastric (stomach) ulcers. Which leads to...

2. Decrease in ADH production, which then causes alcohol to be absorbed directly into the blood stream.

3. A slowing of gastric or stomach emptying which interferes with the esophageal sphincter.

The combination of these can lead to different types of problems including peptic ulcers:

1. The alcohol damaged stomach lining can't make ADH so it **can't block the alcohol from being absorbed directly into the brain,** *damaging the brain.*

2. The slower emptying of the stomach means **the acid stays longer in the stomach**. This causes more damage to the stomach's capillaries leading to *more erosion of the stomach lining.*

3. The esophageal sphincter closes the stomach off from the esophagus. When this is damaged, the acid content in the stomach can reflux back up into the esophagus *causing lesions,* or ulcers there too. Heavy drinkers have higher rates of esophageal cancers and gastric carcinomas.

Alcohol then moves into the intestines.

The Intestines

Heavy alcohol consumption causes damage to the structure and function of the small intestines. There are two main problems:

1. The intestinal lining (mucosa) is composed of microscopic finger-like projections called villi. These villi are full of capillaries necessary to absorb nutrients and release enzymes for digestion. **Alcohol damages and flattens these villi.** *As a result, there is less surface area for absorption of nutrients, inhibition of certain enzymes necessary to transport sugars and proteins into the blood.* In addition, the intestinal cells become damaged and allow the flow of large molecules, like fats, into the blood, which may lead to *gallstones.*

2. Heavy alcohol consumption also *causes problems with peristalsis,* the intestinal muscular contractions which move the food along the intestines. This is probably due to the damage of the nerves along the lining.

The combination of the above leads to major problems with absorption and metabolism, and is a major factor in the malnutrition and ulcerations associated with alcoholism.

Alcohol is then absorbed into the blood stream where it affects the liver and pancreas.

The Pancreas

The Pancreas is a long gland behind the stomach which is crucial to digestion. It secretes enzymes into the small intestines to break down carbohydrates, fats, and proteins so they can be absorbed. The pancreas maintains blood sugar levels by producing insulin and glycogen.

Heavy consumption of alcohol does two things:

1. It irritates the pancreatic duct which pours the digestive enzymes from the pancreas to the small intestine, *causing obstructions in the duct.*

2. Alcohol also **stimulates the pancreas** to make more enzymes to break down the alcohol. Because these enzymes are **activated but blocked** from entering the small intestine, **the pancreas digests itself,** *causing death to tissue.*

This is one of the causes of pancreatitis, inflammation of the pancreas. Pancreatitis usually appears 5 to 10 years after **heavy** drinking. It's symptoms are severe abdominal pain, nausea and vomiting, fever, and tachycardia (increased heart rate). Most people with pancreatitis will recover if they quit drinking, although they may still occasionally have a few bouts of abdominal pain. Twenty percent of people with pancreatitis will experience major complications and five percent will die.

There is also evidence that heavy consumption of alcohol may damage the pancreatic tissue directly. It is probably the highly toxic acetaldehyde from the alcohol breakdown which causes direct damage to the cells. It is not yet known how this may relate to the development of adult onset diabetes, although the two are related.

Women develop pancreatitis more rapidly than men.

The Liver

The liver is the largest organ in the body and provides functions essential to life:

Filtering circulating blood, secreting bile into the GI tract, making proteins and other compounds vital to sustaining life.

The liver is the primary organ for alcohol metabolism. When alcohol reaches the liver, it is broken down into acetaldehyde which is extremely toxic to the liver. Because it is so toxic, acetaldehyde is rapidly converted to acetic acid (vinegar) which is further converted to H_20 and CO_2. While there are other toxic aspects of alcohol in the liver, this large buildup of acetaldehyde associated with heavy drinking is the most understood medical problem.

Research shows that alcohol damages the liver in primarily two ways:

1. Acetaldehyde itself is toxic to the liver and *damages the cells.*

2. When alcohol is ingested, large amounts of oxygen in the liver are diverted from other areas of the liver to metabolize the alcohol. These oxygen deprived areas in the liver can't do their job, part of which is to break down fats, *so the liver becomes fatty.*

There are three types of liver damage: **fatty liver** (just discussed), **alcoholic hepatitis,** and **cirrhosis.**

1. **Fatty liver** is very common among alcoholics - 90 to 100 percent of heavy drinkers show evidence of this. Should the alcoholic quit drinking, this will usually reverse itself in time.

2. **Alcoholic hepatitis** - "Hepa" means liver, "itis" means inflammation, so alcoholic hepatitis means inflammation of the liver cells caused by alcohol. This is a serious condition. *It means that the liver cells are becoming damaged to the point of death.*

   There are varying degrees of alcoholic hepatitis, from mild to fatal. Having alcoholic hepatitis indicates that the person is in middle to end stage alcoholism. When drinking is stopped, the inflammation is reversible. However, any scarring caused by the dead liver cells is permanent.

   Jaundice is a condition caused by alcoholic hepatitis or cirrhosis. Jaundice is the accumulation of bile in the bloodstream, creating a yellow tinge in the eye and skin and an orange tinge in the urine.

   Abnormal blood liver lab values indicate damage to the liver cells. Ten to 35 percent of heavy drinkers will develop alcoholic hepatitis.

3. **Cirrhosis** - In 1989, cirrhosis was the **ninth** leading cause of death in the USA. It is caused by the death of liver cells and scar tissue throughout the liver. **It is an extremely serious condition.**

   The amount, type, pattern of drinking and the person's genetics probably affect the onset of cirrhosis. While it used to be believed that people progressed from fatty liver to alcohol hepatitis to cirrhosis, there is plenty of evidence that many people progress from fatty liver straight to cirrhosis.

Cirrhosis is irreversible. With abstinence, the formation of new scar tissue subsides. Life expectancy depends upon the extent of the cirrhosis. It is suggested that those diagnosed with cirrhosis who continue to drink should say good-bye to their friends and write their wills.

From the liver, alcohol moves through the portal veins into the heart.

Effects on the Heart

Alcohol has a toxic effect on the heart muscle tissue. It causes complex biochemical changes resulting in **increased fat** and **decreased oxygen** in the heart tissue, this essentially affects the heart in two ways:

1. It can affect the heart tissue itself, causing a condition called cardiomyopathy (or degeneration of the heart muscle). This causes an **enlarged** heart with **weaker** contracting muscles.

2. It can cause cardiac arrhythmias - **irregular heartbeats.**

A **weak fatty heart** combined with a **loss of oxygen** and **irregular heartbeats** leads to **heart attacks, heart failure,** and **strokes.** Alcohol induced cardiomyopathy is reversible with abstinence in only about 30 percent of patients. Up to half of the deaths among alcoholics are related to cardiac disease.

From here, the alcohol moves into the cardiovascular system:

The Vascular System

Alcohol causes **hypertension.** Three to four drinks per day will **elevate blood pressure** which leads to **strokes.** In addition, alcohol also affects magnesium levels in the brain causing **brain blood vessel spasms.** This is also a fatal combination. The spasms lead to more hypertension in the brain, **busting vessels** and causing strokes. Hypertension is simply increased pressure in the blood vessels. **When the liver is damaged, the blood can't circulate well.** Blood then backs up in the blood vessels which congests the portal veins in the liver. **Pooling blood** in the portal system, a **weakened heart,** and **hypertension** from drinking adds incredible pressure to those damaged veins, causing them to finally **burst and explode**. An example of this is *esophageal varixes*. As discussed earlier, chronic drinking damages the esophagus and weakens its blood vessels. This weakened vessel becomes "varicosed"; increased pressure backing up in the liver leads to increased pressure in the esophageal vein. This **increased pressure actually causes this vein to explode** and the person usually bleeds to death in a few minutes. *Abstinence can't reverse the varicosed vein, but it will lower the blood pressure and prolong life.*

From the veins, alcohol is directed to the bone marrow, brain, kidneys, and genital organs.

The Blood & Immune System

Alcohol is **toxic to bone marrow**. Basically, it interferes with the formation of red blood cells, causing "immature" cells to be developed instead of healthy red blood cells.

These **immature red blood cells** don't carry oxygen well, and **anemia** also results. In addition, alcohol destroys blood **platelets** which help the blood clot. **Excessive bleeding** and hemorrhages are common in alcoholics.

Alcohol affects the immune system by altering the production and function of many of the **"white cells"**, greatly reducing their ability to fight off infections. As a result, alcoholics *"get sicker faster and stay sicker longer"*. Also, due to high risk behavior by reduced inhibitions, **alcoholics risk higher exposure to the HIV virus.** Because alcohol lowers the immune system, alcoholics are more prone to being infected when exposed.

Endocrine And Reproductive System

Alcohol affects every endocrine organ. How this happens is still not clear, but chronic alcoholics show changes in their **thyroid gland** (which controls, among other things, the basal metabolic rate for the body). Alcohol affects the **adrenal glands** which are responsible for production of **steroids** and **adrenaline** which help us respond to stress and infection. It also affects the **pituitary gland,** the "master" gland which sends messages to these glands.

Alcohol affects the **reproductive system.** Very common among alcoholic men are disorders stemming from alcohol - **impotence, low testosterone levels, low sperm count, and testicular atrophy** or shrinkage. Alcohol seems to affect women's reproduction functions. Pathological **ovary changes, amenorrhea** (absence or sparse menstruation) and problems with **ovulation** are a few of the problems. Because alcohol suppresses hormone secretion, women alcoholics seem to have an earlier onset of menopause as well.

The Brain And Neurological System

1. Alcohol affects the brain and neurological system **directly** and **indirectly.**

2. Heavy drinking **directly** affects brain tissue - obvious examples are **black-outs, hallucinations,** and **seizures.**

3. Alcohol directly affects the brain by **causing change and deterioration** in the brain cells.

4. Alcohol **indirectly** affects the brain by causing damage to the other body organs which help the brain function normally, like the liver and heart.

Prolonged use of alcohol (5 to 10 years) begins to cause damage which affects the structure of the brain and nervous system. The brain is responsible for not only governing the body's function, but is also the center for "human" functions - thinking, feeling, emotions, memory, etc. Even minor damage to the brain can have a major impact on a person's life.

Fifty to seventy percent of detoxed alcoholics show **brain impairment: memory, problem solving, coordination, perception,** and **behavioral changes.** Some of this is reversible with abstinence. *The more severe the drinking and the progression of the disease, the more structural changes happen in the brain and nervous system.*

Periperipheral neuropathy is a condition where nerve endings are damaged, *causing numbness or tingling in fingers and toes.*

A CT Scan of a chronic alcoholic's brain shows **shrinkage** in all areas of the brain, which is irreversible and indicates much more **severe impairment**. Eventually this brain impairment develops into "organic brain syndrome" or "wet brain". There are two organic brain syndromes - **alcoholic dementia** and **Korsakoff's psychosis.** These individuals require constant care - twenty percent of mental institutions house these people at this stage of the disease.

HANDOUT #6

WHEN COMPLETED, THE BLACKBOARD SHOULD LOOK LIKE THIS:

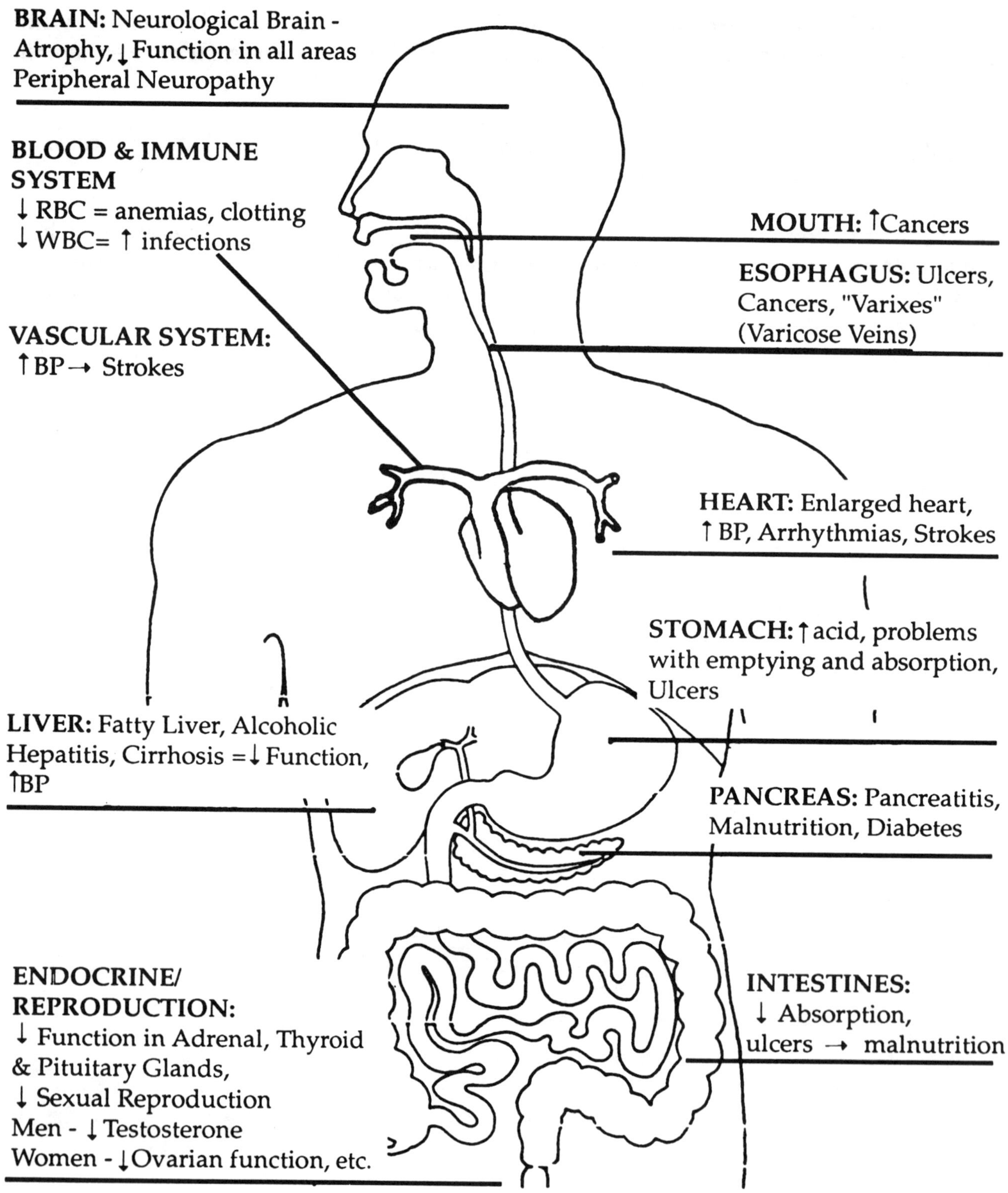

MEDICAL LECTURE FOLLOW-UP GROUPS

There are a variety of ways to follow-up the Medical Aspects of the lecture:

GROUP #1

If you did the sociogram warm-up, do a sociogram follow-up:

Go down the list of the ten body systems affected, having your clients get up and stand together if they have had any of those consequences and make a statement.

Example 1. *"People who've had mouth or esophageal problems stand here. Okay. Mary, make one statement about it."*

Example 2. *"People with stomach problems stand here, make a statement."* Statements should be short. *"I've had burning in my stomach for three years"*, etc.

If you want the group to be deeper, have them attach a feeling to the statement, i.e., *"I've had burning in my stomach for four years. I'm **ashamed** to tell you or I'm **afraid** of the damage I've done,"* etc.

You will find that many people will be in at least half of the different organ system groups.

GROUP #2

Another form of the sociogram is doing a line. Have your clients line up, shoulder to shoulder, from the most affected to the least affected.

1. Do they agree with their positions? (Look at their denial).

2. Have each person make a statement about how they feel in their respective positions.

3. Have the most affected person make a statement to the least affected and vice versa.

GROUP #3

See Handout #7, on the following page, Medical Group # 3

Give the group twenty minutes to fill out the handout.

Then ask them to rejoin in a circle and share their handouts with each other.

Have each person in turn answer their #1 response.

Then going around, have each person answer #2, etc.

Does the group agree or disagree after each person's response?

Close the group with each member making a statement about:

1. What stage of the disease they are in.

2. What's changed for them since the lecture.

There are usually two tricks to doing this group.

1. Most clients get a little rattled after this lecture. There is a tendency for them to want to process their feelings and turn the group into group therapy. It is important to acknowledge their feelings and tell them they there will be a group therapy session later that day to process their feelings. The information **should** be disturbing to those working through denial. *It's okay if not everyone is happy and peaceful when the group ends.*

2. Some will be in total denial about their physical statements. If these people are resistant to treatment in general, **avoid power struggles.** Simply acknowledge their responses and move on. Later, bring up their behavior in the follow-up group therapy. For those with denial but who are also motivated in treatment, ask if you can add your observations about their physical conditions and let them add it to their list.

A variation of a "game" with this is to have the group reconvene. Before reading their handouts, pass around two blank papers per person. Secretly, have each person write what they think the worst consequence is to the person on their left, and on the other sheet, the worst consequence for the person on their right. After the client reads #11 on the handout, have the two people next to them hold their own sheets up. *It provides them with feedback about how others see them.*

Look at discrepancies and process for a minute. Then move on to the next person, etc.

HANDOUT # 7

MEDICAL HANDOUT - Group # 3

The way my body has been affected by alcohol:

1. Mouth & Esophagus:

2. Stomach:

3. Intestines:

4. Pancreas:

5. Liver:

6. Heart:

7. Vascular System:

8. Blood And Immune System:

9. Endocrine And Reproduction:

10. Brain And Neurological:

11. The Worse Physical Consequence To Me Is:

GROUP #4

Always have a follow-up group therapy after this lecture. As mentioned earlier, this lecture will loosen up denial. When denial is loosened, all sorts of underlying feelings will spill out, primarily, shame, anger, grief and loss, and relief. Focus the group on allowing each member to share what happened to them **on an emotional level** during the lecture.

Reinforce the Step 1 concept - that this is about powerlessness - that *"I'm powerless over alcohol and my alcoholism, and when my body is triggered, I have no control over what happens to it. The disease takes its course because that's how it works"*.

Step 1 for most of us is about reaching an emotional or spiritual place with our diseases, finally seeing it and feeling it. Denial is about not having any feelings about our alcoholism. So when your clients are having feelings about their disease, hook them into Step 1 - *"Your **powerlessness** feels like anger to you, or shame to you."*

Reinforce the positive, *"I'm glad you're angry, you're now in recovery"*. **Their physical consequences are examples of unmanageabililty. It's important that they understand how healthy these feelings are as the feelings will move them to a place of accepting the need to change,** then the rest of the Steps fall into place.

Do a follow-up group with this group checking in with them the next day.

Also, give them assignments to share their medical lecture feelings in AA or with their friend, family, or a new group member.

TROUBLE SHOOTING FOR THE DISEASE CONCEPT AND MEDICAL ASPECT LECTURES

WORKING WITH RESISTANCE:

The 70-year-old, 80-pound, emaciated, cirrhotic man with 20 IVs and a feeding tube admitted for alcohol seizures always says, *"I'm fine. My condition is related to an old war injury."* It is the same with court-ordered or family-ordered people. For whatever reasons, accept that they need their denial. Heavy and direct confrontation with these people has two effects:

1. **Equal force exerts equal force**. You push, they push back equally hard. Even if you can finally get them to agree with you, internally, they really don't agree with you. An unspoken stalemate always results, plus now they are angry, and hating you becomes the focus of the rest of their treatment. Steer yourself and the group members away from wanting to jump these folks.

2. **Heavy confrontation may have disastrous emotional consequences.** Again, clients keep their denial to protect themselves from reality. There is no way of knowing what type of ego structure, pathology, and coping skills the person has under their denial. Surgeons don't cut into bodies without knowing where the blood vessels are and how to stop the flow.

   Picture the person sitting on a manhole cover. The manhole cover is their denial and they are keeping this lid on the sewer underneath (seeing their alcoholism). Unless you are the type of therapist or facility that specializes in dealing with blown off manhole covers and spewing emotional guts, use a different tactic than direct blasting. There is no way of knowing what they need to keep repressed.

   Respect and honor their need to keep their denial **for a while**. Usually, denial covers and protects the individual from experiencing their shame. Longer exposure to the treatment process allows the individual to slowly open their lid when they begin to feel safer and have developed better skills for experiencing this shame.

TACTICS FOR DEALING WITH DENIAL:

If it's a group situation, the group eventually responds to a client's adamant denial with anger, disgust or indifference. The client with the denial senses this, anticipates some attack from the group and prepares to defend himself. It is important to defuse and de-escalate your group.

This can be very simple: Most people in group try to model themselves after their therapist. If the therapist is angry with a patient, the group can be angry. If the therapist is gentle and accepting, the group will follow the example.

Simply present your dilemma to the resistant client.

Example: *"For some reason you have a lot of denial about your alcoholism. I get an image of you sitting on a manhole cover."* (Describe this or some other metaphor they can identify with.) *"It's not my job to blow you off your cover or damage you, just to support you when you're ready to begin to peek under the lid like the rest of your peers. Does this make sense to you?"* Ask the group if they see the same thing and are they willing to let Mr. "I'm Only Here For Anxiety" or Miss "My Husband Is My Only Problem" sit on their lid for a little while, by explaining why some people have this need for denial.

Keep processing with group clients until **they** are less reactive to "Mr. Denial". Directing questions to the group about their struggles with the same issue also changes the tone. *"Has anyone else been in this position? Who can relate to Mr. Denial? What was it like for you?"* Now Mr. Denial is not the "target" anymore and has the opportunity to see that his behavior is normal and acceptable (for a while), and the group can empathize and accept Mr. Denial.

Obviously, Mr. Denial cannot stay in treatment just for old war injuries and if his drinking and using is fine. This has to be explained to him and the group. Follow-up groups should focus on the need for such intense **denial** (not the actual alcoholism).

The Denial Lecture also helps them understand what their denial is about.

Explore what their denial protects them from. To do this, play around with different concepts:

1. *"If I was an alcoholic it would mean I'm ________________."*
2. *"I grew up believing alcoholism was ____________________."*
3. *"Saying I was an alcoholic would ______________________."*

Each time the client responds, reinforce their ability to share in groups and be part of it. Compliment them on being able to be "confronted" and still stay in group. Find something good they did in group and let them know that you noticed it.

A good approach for "Mr. Total and Complete Denial I Have Cirrhosis From Too Many Eggs," is to have him explain to you about his level of denial.

Example: *"You have excellent denial around your drinking. When will **you** know that you're becoming physically sick from **alcohol** (not eggs and other things)?"*

These clients usually state some end stage disorder. The goal is not to have them magically accept their disease this instant, but to simply shift their position a baby step closer to recovery and away from their rigid resistance.

Always join with them instead of engaging in a power struggle. They are better at power struggling than you! (Accept this! Look how sick they are! They are very good at not looking at their alcoholism!) If they say *"I'll know I'm sick from drinking when I'm dead,"* (a common response), agree with them: *"Yes, I think this may be the case."*

Ask the group, *"What percentage of people with alcoholism die from alcoholism? Ninety percent. You're probably right, since you are not dead yet, what is the end stage complication of death?"* See the scaling questions technique. Have **him** answer (organic brain, etc.). *"So what symptoms will you have* (memory loss, etc.)?" Have him respond. *"So you're telling me that if you notice problems with memory you'll know your drinking is a problem. Okay, good."*

If they'll know it's a problem when they have cirrhosis or turn yellow, do the same thing. *"Well, you might die by then, what's the stage before it? So, do you think you'll recognize it when you have the shakes or burning in your stomach"*, etc.

Now leave it and move on. **The goal is simply to have them shift their position**, not get rid of their denial today.

Follow-up to their denial can be done in their Steps or other formats. Keep a huge sign posted somewhere which says, **"Whether you like it or not, you have permission to change your mind."** If they mention some new symptom like they had the shakes, point to the sign and say *"Oh my God, you're not changing your mind are you?"* Use humor, share how you've done the same thing, congratulate them.

These are tough people. Anyone with such intense resistance usually has some underlying personality disorder. The above type of work is usually done with personality disordered people. You've performed a miracle if they can shift their position, if you avoided power struggles, if you got the group to agree not to kill him!

THE TWENTY QUESTIONS

Objective: To reinforce recognition of the individual's signs and symptoms of alcoholism. To recognize the commonality of symptoms with other alcoholics.

Materials needed: Blackboard, Twenty Questions Handout, pencils.

Introduction:

Being clear as to whether you are alcoholic or not is the single most important first step to recovery. There may be members in the group who have doubts about whether or not they are real alcoholics or addicts. The signs and symptoms of the disease are scientifically clear.

If you are in a treatment program for chemical dependency, you are probably not there by some freak accident or mistaken case of identity. Cases in which people are misdiagnosed are extremely rare. The diagnosis is relatively easy to make.

The problem lies in the alcoholic's ability to recognize it. Some of us know we are alcoholics before we get sober and many of us, when we are out there using, do not have a clue (this is our denial). For all of us, it appears that to clearly see the impact of our disease, we need to stop using and be willing to see the truth.

The following simple exercise describes some of the signs and symptoms of chemical dependency. Please complete it as honestly as you can.

Directions:

Pass out the Twenty Questions Handout and pencils.
Allow 10 to 15 minutes for completion.
Number 1 through 20 on the blackboard.
Ask a group member to be a secretary.
Read each question individually going around the group. After each question, ask the group by a show of hands how many members answered yes to each question.
Ask clients for a few specific examples of how the statement applies to them.
Have the secretary add the numbers and record them next to the appropriate number on the blackboard.

The results should show that we have a group of real alcoholics in our midst! Ask if any one in the group has doubts about whether they have the disease. If yes, ask the client what the group can do to help move him through the doubt.

Example: *"Can we help by pointing out any signs and symptoms that you bring up in groups?"*

End the group with some joining exercise. Congratulate participants on their progress in breaking through denial.

Example: *"It looks like we are all in this together. Let's join hands and say the "Serenity Prayer."*

Note: This group is not a processing group. It will work well with dual diagnoses clients due to its simplicity and non-threatening format.

HANDOUT # 8

TWENTY QUESTIONS
ARE YOU AN ALCOHOLIC?

Answer **Yes** or **No** to each question

1. Do you lose time from work due to drinking? __________
2. Is drinking/using making your home life unhappy? __________
3. Do you drink/use because you are shy with other people? __________
4. Is drinking/using affecting your reputation? __________
5. Have you ever felt remorse after drinking/using? __________
6. Have you gotten into financial difficulties as a result of drinking/using? __________
7. Do you turn to lower companions and an inferior environment when drinking? __________
8. Does your drinking/using make you careless of your family's welfare? __________
9. Has your ambition decreased since you started drinking/using? __________
10. Do you crave a drink or drug at a definite time daily? __________

11. Do you want a drink or drug the next morning? ___________

12. Does drinking/using cause you to have difficulty sleeping? ___________

13. Has your efficiency decreased since you started drinking/using? ___________

14. Is drinking/using jeopardizing your job or business? ___________

15. Do you drink/use to escape from worries or trouble? ___________

16. Do you drink/use alone? ___________

17. Have you ever had a complete loss of memory as a result of drinking/using? ___________

18. Has your physician ever treated you for drinking/using? ___________

19. Do you drink/use to build up your self-confidence? ___________

20. Have you ever been to a hospital or institution on account of drinking/using? ___________

If you have answered Yes to any **one** of these questions, this is a definite warning that you may be an alcoholic.

If you have answered Yes to any **two**, the chances are that you are an alcoholic.

If you have answered Yes to **three or more**, you are definitely an alcoholic.

DENIAL

"We have troubles because we refuse to grow up," said the Master. *"How will we know when we have grown up?"*, asked the student. *"When we no longer need to be lied to."*

Being in recovery means we don't need or want to lie to ourselves. Denial is our escape from reality, our fantasy. It's lying to ourselves. All is fine, and we are in control. Denial keeps us from the truth. **A spiritual reality is that when we experience truth, we can change and transform.**

Many of us feel that our disease has its own personality and voice. We all have different parts or aspects to our personality. For example, most of us feel and behave differently at work than when we are with our parents, around our kids, on a hot date, or in a classroom. We tell our kids not to lie and mean it, then we lie to our boss, the IRS, and our own mothers. It is as if we have different and real personalities existing in our consciousness. The disease also has a life of its own and its own voice. To stay "alive," it creates its own story to tell us. Essentially, it tells us we are fine and do not have the disease so we can keep using. This untrue story that we hear is our denial.

To recover from chemical dependency, we need to know how our disease lies to us, and how **we lie to ourselves**. We bring the truth in so we can have a chance to change our broken lives. When we go to 12 Step meetings, we will often hear people talk about what "their disease is saying": *"My disease wants me to go to my using friends house, my disease thinks that one beer won't hurt me."* These people are familiar with their denial and how it works in them.

Denial is a protective mechanism. It is a defense. It keeps us from **feeling** the painful and uncomfortable truth about both our powerlessness and the consequences or unmanageability of our addictions. If we cannot feel or see these consequences, everything is fine and our disease can stay alive and active.

Denial comes in many forms. It is not just for chemical dependents either. If you are human, you have denial about something - your relationships, your behavior, your health, your family, etc. We all want everything to "be fine." We have denial to protect us from pain.

As chemical dependents, to keep our denial is to die. In the process, we create pain for those around us. We have denial about this too. To recover, we need to see our denial and see how it works so that we can loosen the grip of our addictions. Denial is replaced by the truth and acceptance.

To be in denial feels like anger, fear, shame, and isolation. Instead of being cold and cut off from ourselves and others, we can be warm and begin to grow again.

Defenses are the specific way we ward off attacks to our denial. Some defenses are conscious and we are aware of them. Others are subconscious. We use both to keep our denial intact.

Listed below are common defenses, or forms of denial. We use all forms of denial, although there are some that become our favorites.

1. **Simple denial -** Simply denying being chemically dependent. Example: *"You're an alcoholic." "No, I'm not."*

2. **Minimizing -** This is about making our chemical dependency or using seem less. Example: *"Yes, I drink, but not that much." "I wasn't that bad at the party."*

3. **Rationalizing -** Making excuses about our using. Example: *"I can't sleep, so I drink or take pills." "I need narcotics for my bad back." "I had a bad day."*

4. **Blaming -** Using because we "had to." Something "made us." The responsibility lies somewhere else, not with us. Example: *"If my wife was nicer, I wouldn't need to drink!" "I lost my job, that's what made me drink."*

5. **Bargaining -** Cutting deals. Example: *"I'll quit if you quit smoking." "I'll quit when there's less stress at work."*

6. **Intellectualizing or Generalizing** - Using theories about your chemical dependency, keeping it general and vague. Example: *"My family is alcoholic and I have the wrong genes." "My childhood was so bad, it's a way of coping with my underlying feelings."*

7. **Diversion** - Changing the subject. Example: *"Yeah I got drunk last night, so what's for dinner?"* or *"My drinking bothers you? Your weight bothers me!"*

8. **Passivity - Ignoring it or being a victim.** Example: *"I've tried to quit, but it's stronger than me." "There's nothing I can do." "If I only had more willpower...."*

9. **Hostility -** Scaring or threatening people away from discussing it. Example: *"I'm lousy in bed when I'm drunk? Fine, no more sex." "Get off my back!" "You like my paychecks, don't you?"*

FACILITATING THE DENIAL GROUP

Materials needed: Blackboard, Handout #9 and #10.

The easiest way to begin the group is to have the group discuss what denial is and the types of denial. Using a blackboard, have somebody list what the members say. Let them brainstorm for a while.

Pass out the **Denial Lecture, Handout # 9.** Let each member read a paragraph, comment, and move on. Encourage group discussions throughout the reading. Encourage examples from the group. At the end, pass out the remaining handouts. Provide about one hour to complete the work. Rejoin.

Let person A read their Page 1, "My denial around drinking and using."

Have person A stop after each example to see if the group agrees with their denial until that page is complete. A simple "thumbs up" or "thumbs down" from the group will work.

Then have person B read their Page 1. Depending upon the needs of the group, keep it light or use it as a time for confrontation. Compliment them on seeing their denial.

In the same fashion, do Pages 2 and 3. Have each person sum up their most difficult area of denial and how they plan to work with it.

HANDOUT # 10

DENIAL

In the next three sections, look at how your denial works in three areas: Your disease, the effect on your family (or relationship, **if you don't have a family**), and your need to work a recovery program like AA.
Give a specific example for each:

The ways I have denial around my drinking/using:

1. **Simple denial**

2. **Minimizing**

3. **Rationalizing**

4. **Blaming**

5. **Bargaining**

6. **Intellectualizing**

7. **Diversion**

8. **Passivity**

9. **Hostility**

Place a ✓ next to your favorite denial.
Place a * next to the ones you had the most difficulty with. A * means that you still have excellent denial about your denial.

My denial about how my drinking/using has affected my family. Give specific examples.

1. **Simple denial**

2. **Minimizing**

3. **Rationalizing**

4. **Blaming**

5. **Bargaining**

6. **Intellectualizing**

7. **Diversion**

8. **Passivity**

9. **Hostility**

Place a ✓ next to your favorite denial.
Place a * next to the ones you had the most difficulty with. A * means that you still have excellent denial about your denial.

My denial about working a program.
Give specific examples.

1. **Simple denial**

2. **Minimizing**

3. **Rationalizing**

4. **Blaming**

5. **Bargaining**

6. **Intellectualizing**

7. **Diversion**

8. **Passivity**

9. **Hostility**

Place a ✓ next to your favorite denial.
Place a * next to the ones you had the most difficulty with. A * means that you still have excellent denial about your denial.

FOOD, THE MIND ALTERING DRUG

Until recently, nutrition has been all but ignored in treatment centers. What makes this alarming is that poor nutrition is most likely **the leading cause of relapse**. Most treatment centers do not understand this. Warnings may be given about too much sugar or caffeine with hollow explanations, no formal education, and no dietary plan or follow-up for relapse prevention.

Nutrition is **the most crucial factor** in the client's ability to maintain sobriety. Imagine giving your clients an open prescription for amphetamines and tranquilizers, instructing them to take different combinations of them 20 times per day, and then deal with the stressors of new sobriety. This is precisely what we are doing when we do not educate our clients about the other mind and emotionally altering use of addictive chemicals — food.

As clinicians, some of us have a solid working comprehension of nutrition and chemical dependency. Most of us bring 20 crates of glazed donuts on the unit for special occasions. In regard to nutrition, we all have our different beliefs and practices. The best way to do this lecture is:

1. Read the information in this handout.
2. "Reframe" the information depending upon the functioning level of the group.
3. Integrate it with your own additional comments and stories.

Depending upon your time constraints, this can be one long lecture with discussion, or you can present two shorter lectures by breaking Food and Caffeine into separate groups.

Before giving your lecture, pass around the handout, "Yesterday's Diet."

There are three primary focuses which need to be discussed in a nutrition/relapse prevention lecture.

1. The effects of sugar and processed foods on the chemically dependent.
2. The effects of caffeine.
3. Developing a recovery food plan. Included throughout this section will be suggestions for presenting the information as well as guidelines for a healthy recovery diet.

THE LECTURE: FOOD, THE MIND ALTERING DRUG

I. To Start: Looking at sugars:

1. **Sugars are addicting.**

2. **Sugars are mind altering.**

1. Sugars are addicting.

This is a statement that needs little explanation. To prove your point, simply ask the group for volunteers willing to quit using all sugars and processed foods. What would happen to them in 24 hours? They will be cranky, irritable, and have low energy for at least the first day or two. **They will experience sugar withdrawal.**

To explain this concept to clients, use the general addiction theory that: To be an addictive substance, something needs to cause an **altered sensorium, tolerance** and **withdrawal**.

These three examples prove the point about addiction:

Give your 5-year-old three candy bars and they will get "wired" and race around, become angry or aggressive, irritable, and then they will "crash." Their mind is **altered**.

One hundred years ago, we ate five to ten pounds of sugar per person. Today, in the USA, the average person consumes 115 to 150 pounds of sugar per person. Sugar is in much of the "store bought" foods that we eat such as: Bread, canned foods, spaghetti sauces and McDonald's fries. We have developed **tolerance**.

Eliminate all sugars from the average diet and the person will experience **withdrawal** (mentioned above) and **craving**.

2. Sugars are mind altering.

To understand this, we need a little background on hypoglycemia, more specifically, the condition called **functional hypoglycemia.** There are literally thousands of studies on hypoglycemia. To keep it simple, the following explains the general idea. First, keep in mind that 90 to 100% of alcoholics are functional hypoglycemics. (This is explained later.)

The origins of hypoglycemia are complicated and blood sugar levels are affected by numerous factors and conditions. To generalize and oversimplify, this is what happens:

Sugar enters the blood stream and is regulated by two hormones produced in the pancreas, insulin and glucagon.

When **too much sugar is in the blood, insulin** is released into the blood stream to lower the blood sugar levels. **Insulin removes sugars** from the blood by moving the sugars into the body's cells where it can be used for the cell's energy. These excess sugars are converted to glycogen in the liver for storage or into fats. When the body cannot make any or enough insulin, the sugar remains in the blood which is the condition known as diabetes.

Conversely, **when the blood is low on sugar,** meaning that the cells in the body do not have the food they need, the other pancreatic hormone, **glucagon,** tells the liver to break down its stored sugars (glycogen) and **release the sugars back into the blood** to circulate. This is essentially how the body remains in sugar balance.

Since all sugars bathe the brain, **too much sugar** in the blood has **harmful physical** and **emotional** effects. The emotional effects of *hyperglycemia* (hyper=too much, glycemia=sugar) can be devastating. Again, picture the 5-year-old with three candy bars, what happens from too much sugar **emotionally** for this little tyke? The same thing happens in adults. Initially, the body feels "good" and energized by adding sugar. However, **when we keep adding more sugar,** the central nervous system becomes **more stimulated** and this is experienced both physically and emotionally.

Draw this diagram on the blackboard:

EMOTIONAL EFFECTS OF TOO MUCH SUGAR:

Death

Coma

Diabetic ranges: { Stupor

Drowsiness

Anxiety

Anger

Agitation

Elevating effects: { Irritability

Too Energetic, Hyperactive

Feeling "Good", Energetic

NORMAL SUGAR LEVEL

Too **little** blood sugar can result from fasting, but low blood sugar is **usually** caused by the body's response to **too much sugar.** To protect the brain from coma by a load of sugar that has just been dumped into the blood, like from a donut or alcohol, the pancreas releases **a lot** of insulin. This results in a big surge of insulin which **drops** the sugar level **below normal,** or a *hypoglycemic* state (low blood sugar). Hypoglycemia has its physical and emotional effects as well.

Now add this to your diagram on the blackboard:

EMOTIONAL EFFECTS OF TOO LITTLE SUGAR:

NORMAL SUGAR LEVEL

Low Sugar ↓

Low Energy

Irritability

Frustration

Poor Concentration

Agitation

Anger

Drowsiness

Coma

Death

For the lecture, set your chalkboard up to look like this.

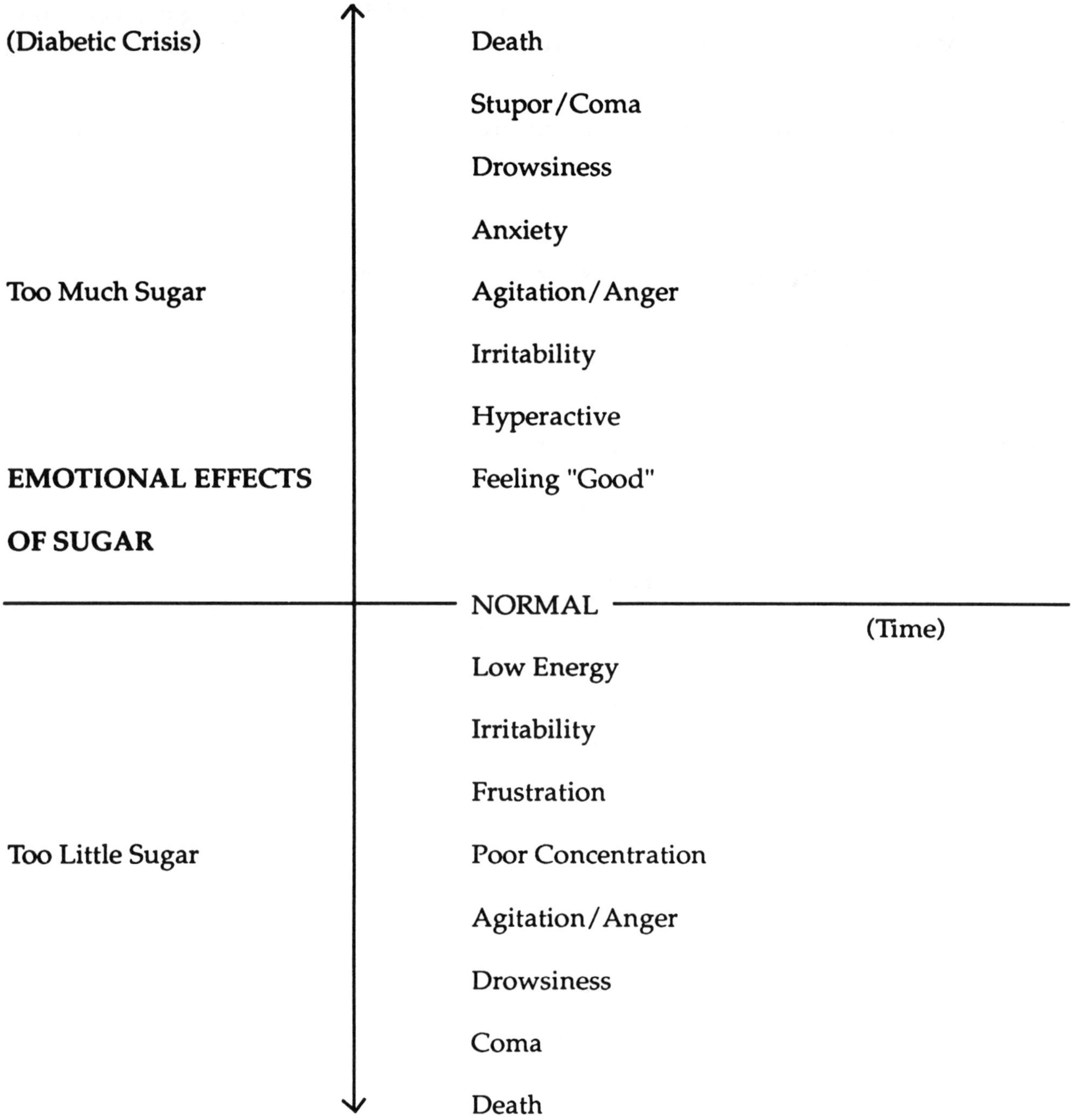

The horizontal axis is now in place in the diagram.

To finish this part of the lecture, the vertical axis "time" line needs to be completed. The "time" line looks at the **amount of time** it takes to experience the mood swings from eating sugar. **To do this, here is the two minute explanation of sugars.**

Sugars are carbohydrates. If they watch television, most clients have heard the terms "simple sugars" and "complex carbohydrates."

All "sugars" are carbohydrates. All plants are carbohydrates.

Types of "sugars" are determined by the **length** of their molecule:

- **Simple** or (sweet) sugars consist of lots of **short** stranded molecules hooked together;
- **Complex** sugars (plant foods) are similar strands of molecules, just hooked into very **long** strands.

All carbohydrates are broken down into a **one molecular** sugar the body can use—**glucose.**

So, the carbohydrate table sugar or **sucrose** (cane sugar), is simply a very short-chained carbohydrate. Because it is such a **small** molecule, it can be digested or broken down into glucose very quickly and **moves into the blood at a very rapid pace**.

The **more complex** the carbohydrate, the **longer** it takes to be broken down into glucose and enter the blood stream. Some carbohydrates are so long that there is never enough time in the intestines to break them down and they pass through the large intestine fairly intact. The cellulose fiber found in "roughage" or "bulk" foods, like the hulls on grains and beans are examples of this.

This is the mechanism which relates to relapse:

For unknown reasons, most alcoholics are functional hypoglycemics ("functional" meaning that their blood sugar levels drop drastically but they can still walk around). For reasons not understood, when the alcoholic eats a **simple** sugar that enters the blood stream rapidly, *the pancreas over reacts.* It **pours** insulin into the blood, quickly dropping the blood sugar level below normal. They "crash." They can feel their energy level dropping and feel the irritation set in.

Like any good alcoholic or addict , when they feel the withdrawal begin, they "fix" again, or eat more sugar. This stops the sugar crash or withdrawal. However, to cope with the next dose of sugar, the pancreas squirts out even more insulin, another crash, more sugar, and so forth. **If they eat table sugars, they can never maintain "normal" blood sugars or mood.** This will not exist for them. They will have mood swings **all day long**.

This directly relates to relapse for two reasons. First, physiologically, these great fluctuations in sugar levels and mood are identical to the sugar levels in drinking. When the blood sugar levels are low, the body needs or "craves" more sugar. Because of the long standing pattern of alcohol abuse, the body craves the sugar it customarily received, alcohol. Drop the blood sugar and the most natural **unconscious** response is to crave the blood sugar that the body is used to — alcohol. Setting up the craving cycle five times per day with sugar leads to drinking. **It is the natural, expected progression.** If I am a candy bar abuser and I kick the habit, I will crave candy bars, not guavas that I have never eaten. ***I will crave my sugar of choice and for alcoholics this means alcohol.***

Also, and of equal importance, if the person is an amphetamine abuser — a cocaine or speed addict — then when **their** blood sugar levels drop, the "pick me up" for this feeling will be cocaine, hence unnecessary cocaine craving. To sum it up, ***when we use the simple carbohydrates of sugars, we set up a constant craving cycle.***

The second factor related to relapse is as follows: When the chemically dependent person starts their day with sugar, they will get high and crash within two to three hours. The fact that it's actually a beautiful day and they won the million dollar lottery does not matter. They are powerless over their blood sugar levels and physiologically based moods. Most people in early recovery do not win the lottery. Instead, their wife is mad, the kids are late for school, and the bills are piling up. So, ***when you combine the swinging and crashing throughout the day from sugar, and add a tablespoon of stress to that, you will be mixing yourself another drink or drug.***

It must be emphasized to clients that the extent and severity of the mood swing depends upon the length of the carbohydrate chain put into the stomach. The shorter the sugar, the more quick and rapid the absorption into the blood. This results in the high feeling. To balance this, there is a resulting, whopping amount of insulin released to protect the brain from stupor resulting in the deeper "crash."

To complete the rest of the diagram, the time line, it is necessary to know a bit about the types of carbohydrates and the amount of time they require to break down in the body.

To review:
A short chained carbohydrate results in quick insulin surges and crashes.
Long chained carbohydrates don't do this as they enter the blood stream slowly. They are like a "time-released pill." Since they enter the blood slowly, the brain and pancreas don't freak out, therefore, there is a slow burn of energy, no highs or lows, and no mood swings. Because I am not physically impaired when I eat long chained carbohydrates, I can handle the stress of life one thing at a time.

TYPES OF SUGARS

Short strand molecules: Table sugar (sucrose)
Processed grains
Processed grains, like white flour, are whole grains which have been "refined," or broken down into small molecules to be "easily digestible." Since they are now a simple sugar, **they will cause mood swings.**

Medium molecules: Fruits
Medium molecules are slower to break down and cause slight elevations in mood. The sweeter the fruit, the more sugar they contain, and the higher the swing. Grapes are a sweet fruit. The less sweet the fruit, the longer the molecular chain. No mood swings are experienced from eating bananas.

Long strand molecules: Grains (Brown rice, whole wheat grains, etc.)
Lentils/Beans
These take four to six hours to burn and cause no mood swings. They are efficient "time-released" energy.

To keep this from being too technical, here is the general idea:

EATING SUGAR VERSUS COMPLEX CARBOHYDRATES:

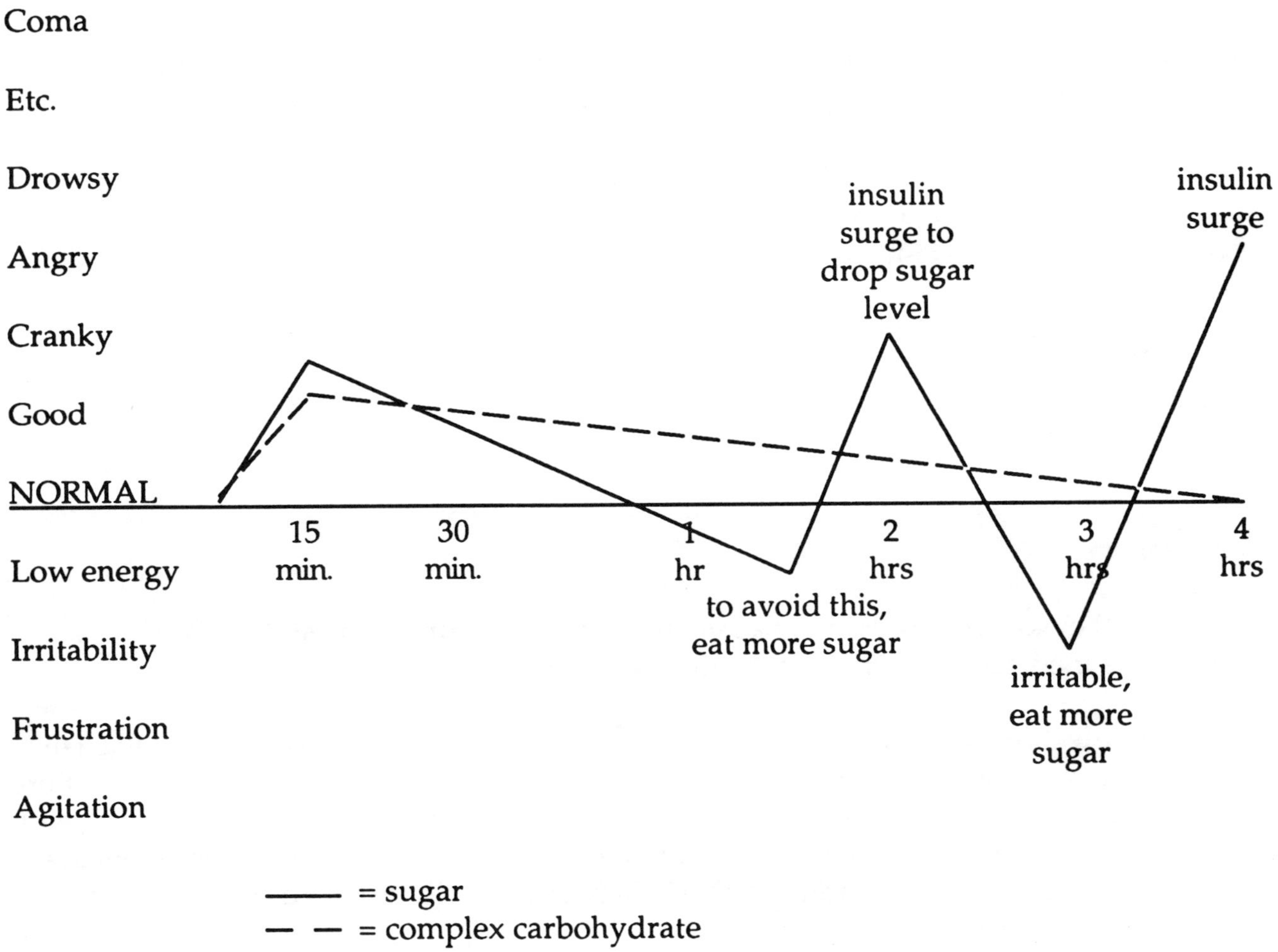

The more sugar they eat, the higher up the scale they climb and the lower they drop. The effects begin in about one-half hour and lasts for two to three hours.

Group follow-up:

#1. Play around with these foods in the group. What is the best diet for recovery?
Answer: No sugar and lots of complex carbohydrates, a hypoglycemic type diet.

List these foods on the board:

Recovering Foods	**Using Foods**
Whole Grain Fruits, Vegetables Honey In Small Amounts	Sugars, Sodas, Syrups White Flour, Pastas Canned Sauces (they contain sugar-dextrose, corn syrup, etc.) Most cereals in a box

A hypoglycemic type of diet also includes foods rich in proteins. Grain and lentil combinations, meats, fish, eggs, milk, cheese and nuts are also "good" foods.

#2. Have the group design a healthy:

Breakfast: Example: Egg and cheese omelet, whole grain bread, milk or "decaf."

Lunch:

Dinner:

Snacks:

When do they know they are in relapse without picking up that first drink?
What does medicating your feelings with food mean?

In the same lecture, using the same graph already on the board, inform the group that if they really want to get totally whacked out and psycho before 10 AM, they should add more amphetamines to their system, like coffee! Oh, what two cups of speed (coffee) laced with 2 tablespoons of more speed (sugar) can do for getting them started on the right foot every day. Who cares if the Stock Market crashes? They can experience their own crash four times in one morning, watching the "Soaps"!

CAFFEINE — THE FAVORITE AMPHETAMINE DRUG

Introduction:

It is important to spend some time discussing caffeine. Most chemically dependent people abuse caffeine to avoid some of the withdrawal symptoms of their active addiction. We use coffee in the morning and all day to ward off the hangover headache and low energy level, and to avoid the cocaine or amphetamine "crash," etc. When *our clients get sober, they will still abuse caffeine, particularly as an attempt to alter their consciousness and physical energy levels.* In early recovery, this is particularly dangerous as the physical effects of caffeine lead to **mood swings, addiction,** and **withdrawal.** With drug induced mood swings affecting their brains and emotions, concentration, and sleep, to name a few, little stressors become huge. This starts your clients off with a major handicap in their recovery which is not necessary.

About Caffeine:

1. Caffeine is an amphetamine or stimulant drug. It is the active ingredient in coffee, tea, and the cola nut. (These are the most common forms of caffeine in the USA.)

2. Caffeine is highly addicting. One develops tolerance to the drug in approximately four days.

3. Caffeine levels peak in the blood about 30 to 60 minutes after ingestion. The half life of caffeine is about 3 hours (meaning that half of the dose is still in the system 3 hours later). It is completely eliminated in the urine by about 12 hours.

4. Smokers metabolize caffeine 50% faster than non-smokers. Caffeine and nicotine have opposite effects on the body. The smoker will feel the effects of caffeine for a shorter period of time, so if addicted to caffeine, they will need to double their doses over the non-smoking caffeine drinker/addict.

5. Pregnancy slows the metabolism of caffeine, therefore, the drug stays much longer in pregnant women and their fetuses.

6. Birth control pills double the effect of caffeine. Women using birth control pills will feel a strong caffeine reaction to their second cup of caffeine.

7. Caffeine is found in saliva, semen, and mother's milk.

Caffeine Content of Standard Beverages

Average Cup of Coffee	80 mg
Strong Cup of Coffee	120 mg
Average Cup of Tea	40 mg
Average Soft Drink (includes diet sodas)	40 mg

For the average man, **caffeine poisoning** occurs after eight cups of strong coffee. The symptoms are:

1. Hyperventilation
2. Tachycardia (rapid heart rate)
3. Convulsions, muscle spasms
4. Ventricular fibrillation
5. Low levels of potassium in the blood
6. Increased levels of sugar, as in the diabetic state

Caffeine withdrawal occurs 3 to 6 hours after the last cup. The symptoms include:

1. Headache
2. Anxiety
3. Fatigue/exhaustion
4. Runny nose
5. Sweating
6. General muscle pains

Chronic use of caffeine leads to:

1. Increased heart disease (increased blood pressure, increased arrhythmias, increased cholesterol).

2. Increased cancer, especially bladder cancer in men.

3. Reproductive problems for women.

One in four adults are addicted to caffeine.
One in thirty adults experience physical consequences directly related to caffeine use — heart disease, cancer, behavioral disorders.

I. Effects On The Brain And Central Nervous System:

The benefits of caffeine are seen with one to two cups of average coffee or tea per day. One to two cups of coffee can prolong the amount of time a person can perform physically exhausting work. It aids endurance. It does not improve the quality of work. Because it is beneficial for physical endurance, in many parts of the world it is given to work animals. It is also banned from the Olympics — athletes are disqualified for positive caffeine drug tests.

Caffeine has negative affects on intelligence. One to two cups increases the attention span or mental alertness. The factory worker will be able to stay on the job longer and feel sharper. However, caffeine worsens short term memory, so the worker will actually make more mistakes. In effect, it speeds up performance at the cost of increased errors.

A major point about caffeine is that caffeine has a severe effect on sleep. Sleep is of crucial importance to the chemically dependent. Most practicing chemical dependents use their drugs to induce sleep. After detox, it will take a few months for their bodies to establish normal sleep cycles. Generally, non-caffeine drinkers require 30 minutes to fall asleep, then sleep for 7.4 hours. After ingesting 1 1/2 cups of coffee, it takes **2** hours to fall asleep and sleep lasts only 5 hours. Also, these caffeine drinkers are more easily roused and are awakened by intense dreams or noises.

If the newly detoxed client abuses coffee, he will experience sleep disturbance from post-withdrawal, compounded by the caffeine induced insomnia. To obtain "good sleep," this situation will induce drug ideation and euphoric recall. ***Caffeine abuse can and will set them up for relapse.***

II. Effects On Other Parts Of The Body:

Caffeine increases acid in the stomach and slows peristalsis in the small intestine. This combination can cause or aggravate ulcers. In addition, it increases large intestine mobility causing diarrhea or excessive water loss.

Lecture Suggestions:

Using the just conveyed "sugar and mood chart" that was put on the board during the first half of the lecture, overlap a separate caffeine line in a different colored chalk. Again, caffeine takes about 30 to 60 minutes to peak in the blood, so if your clients drink two cups of coffee first thing in the morning, then another cup at 10 AM, reflect this in the chart.

Impress upon the client that the mood swings below are how they will feel if they have 2 cups of coffee with sugar!!

EATING SUGAR VERSUS COMPLEX CARBOHYDRATES:

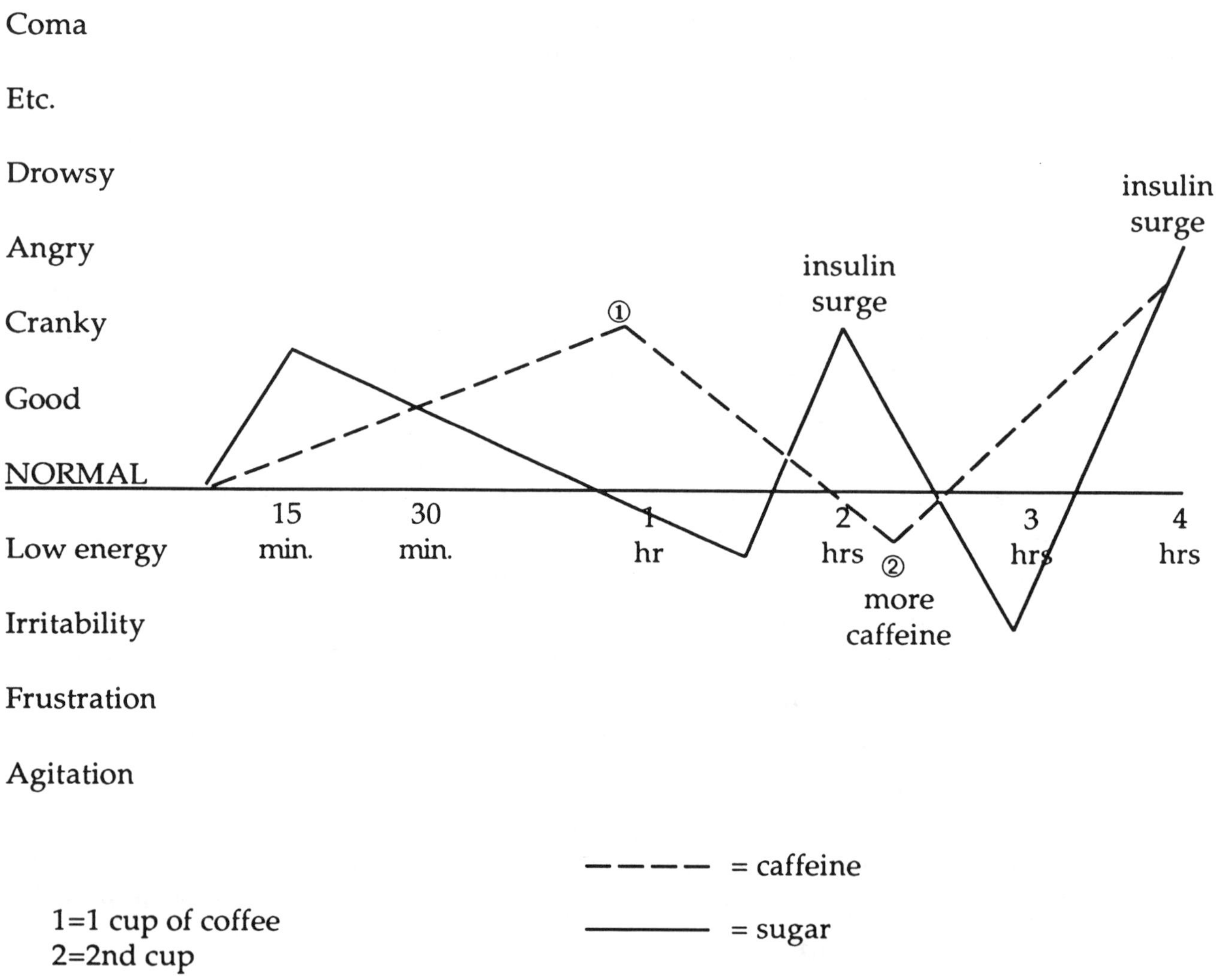

TO KICK THE HABITS: The acute effects of sugar and caffeine withdrawal last approximately 24 hours. Low energy levels may persist for a few days, but the severe headaches and fatigue subside in a day or two. Instruct your clients to choose a day when there is little stress so they can tolerate the withdrawal. Many types of aspirin contain caffeine, so they will need to check the labels. In fact, suggest checking the labels of all of the foods they eat and drink so they can find the hidden sugars, processed ingredients, and caffeine. Many will find that more than half of their "normal" foods are loaded.

The two parts on sugar and caffeine will take about an hour to present. Depending upon the time of your group, process some of the following questions:

Who is addicted to sugars (including white flour, etc.), and caffeine? How?
Who can relate to the mood swings caused by both drugs?
What can you change in your using behavior today? (Refer to their "Yesterday's Diet" Handout #11 and have them make appropriate changes.)

FOLLOW-UP

Depending upon your type of facility, you may request that people not show up "loaded." If you are a day treatment facility, you may notice your clients "nodding" or drowsy in your 10 AM group. Ask them how much sugar they had in their breakfast and how much coffee the day before.

Do not enable their habits, confront them. If they are drugged up in your groups, they will be drugged up at work, as well as experiencing unnecessary craving.

Is diet included in their discharge plan?

HANDOUT # 11

YESTERDAY'S DIET

Take a few minutes to complete this handout. List all the meals, snacks, and drinks that you consumed yesterday. Include the approximate times. Be as specific as possible in describing the types of food that you ate (if you ate bread include whether it was white, whole wheat, etc.). If you drank something, how was it sweetened?

TIME **TYPE OF FOOD OR DRINK**

Notes to Clinicians:

As you know, a good portion of your clients will have active, unresolved conjunctive eating disorders. This lecture will stimulate questions they may have about them. We would like to stress that eating disorders are a primary disease and **need to be addressed as part of the primary treatment.**

There are not many concrete studies about treatment outcomes for these dual addicted people, but outcome trends are beginning to emerge. It is believed that the eating disorder is the **primary disease** - it occurs before the chemical addiction. Substance abuse is the second addiction which happens to get the individual into treatment. Therefore, removing only the active chemical use leaves the primary disease, the eating disorder intact. Untreated, it is still well and alive and will shortly manifest its symptoms again, including the need for chemical use. The dynamic is much more complex than this, but essentially, untreated eating disorders are fatal primary diseases requiring **immediate** treatment.

Untreated, eating disorders will lead back to chemical use as the primary addiction, the eating disorder, is still alive and untreated. Please understand: *A bulemic alcoholic who goes through treatment without her bulemia being treated* ***has not gone through treatment.*** This is a sweeping generalization, but it is generally true.

For us to work up adequate and comprehensive groups on eating disorders would require a separate manual.

Here are some suggestions:

1. Utilize an eating disorder clinical specialist on your team or as a consultant.

2. Develop a staff person to be the unit eating disorder "specialist". Send them to workshops, give them the time they need to develop the necessary skills. Then, let them be the primary counselor for these clients.

3. Always refer eating disordered people to clinical specialists as part of their discharge planning.

4. Include the eating disorder in the Aftercare/Recovery Plan.

5. Develop some affiliation with Overeaters Anonymous. Ask these folks to run a weekly group for you as part of your regular treatment structure. Ask OA for a temporary sponsor list and have your client begin to contact OA soon into treatment.

AIDS AND CHEMICAL DEPENDENCY

Whether by deliberate action or by circumstance, chemical dependency caregivers will find themselves on the front line in the fight against AIDS. We believe no one is better equipped to meet this challenge. No one is more adept at dealing with the denial, stigma, and shame that encompasses alcoholics, other drug addicts, and people with AIDS. No one is more skilled in enlisting family, lovers, friends, employers, and other health professionals to participate in the process of intervention, Twelve Step recovery and relapse prevention.

This presentation will address the connections and similarities between HIV disease and chemical dependency. Do you know what HIV disease is? Do you know how it travels? Do you know what you can do to protect yourself? All of us need to be able to answer yes because AIDS is one of the most serious public health problems being faced by this generation.

Individual Goal: Clients will gain a basic understanding of AIDS and its connection to their chemical dependency. At the end of this presentation they will be able to make an informed choice about testing.

Group Goal: Unity is created as clients learn concepts of stigma and shame. Collective fear, misunderstanding and prejudice around HIV are addressed.

Materials needed: Blackboard. This is Handout #12. It may be distributed after the lecture.

Notes to Clinicians: It is essential to talk simply, clearly, to repeat the message, and to do so in language that the client understands. That does not mean patronizing the clients with phony and affected lingo. It means using whatever language, pictures, gestures, or ideas you need to get the message across. For many of us, it is difficult to talk about sexual behavior with our clients. It is even more difficult to hear them speak of "fucking" and "getting fucked." It takes practice, and sometimes it may help for you to go to lectures by sex therapists or to do role playing with your colleagues.

One exercise you can do with your peers is to brainstorm together, putting all "dirty words" on the board, test questioning techniques with each other, and allow your own problems with the language to be confronted and defused. Actually, this is not much different from learning how to deal with other unpleasant issues, such as death and dying, or cancer in children.

Presentation: Today, we will be talking about AIDS. It is a very serious presentation. It might save your life. Some of you know a great deal about AIDS and HIV disease. For some of you this may be new information. For all of you, there are no stupid questions. If, for any reason, you are unable to ask your question in this group, see me afterward. Another suggestion is to write your question on a piece of paper and give it to me some time today. The information you hear here is **not** confidential. In fact, I encourage you to share it with as many of your friends and relatives as possible. Your personal sharing of your own experience is, however, confidential. It is yours and yours alone.

Before going on, get a pledge of confidentiality from the group.

What Is AIDS?

AIDS stands for **Acquired Immune Deficiency Syndrome**. We are all surrounded by a variety of microorganisms that can make us sick — in the air we breathe, on our pets, in the food we eat. Normally, we are protected from these potential intruders by powerful barriers. The most important first line barriers we have are our skin and the mucous membrane linings of our mouth, rectum, vagina, or penis.

Much like a good football team, the body does not depend on a single line of defense. it has secondary defenders who come into action if the first line breaks down or is penetrated. The most important of these defenders, especially in relation to AIDS, are the blood's T-helper cells.

One type of T cell is called a **CD4 cell.** These are the cells that reject foreign infections and tumors. They are the cells that would reject a transplanted heart or kidney. If these CD4 cells are destroyed, a variety of diseases have the opportunity to take over our bodies. These opportunistic illnesses include pneumonia and cancer among many others. It is these opportunistic infections that cause people to get sick. If someone has an illness because of **the suppression of their T cells**, we say they have AIDS.

The virus that suppresses and destroys the CD4 cells is called HIV. It stands for **Human Immunodeficiency Virus**. If someone has the virus, we say they have HIV disease. The presence of HIV in the blood determines who is at high risk for developing AIDS. It does **not** mean that a person has AIDS. And, just to make matters more confusing, it does **not** mean that the person with HIV in their blood will go on to develop AIDS. The main way HIV is spread among people is through the transmission of HIV-infected blood or semen.

What Does It Look Like?

The following list of symptoms can be present in people regardless of whether they are infected with HIV. However, if any of these symptoms persist, **DON'T IGNORE THEM** -- notify your doctor immediately. Many of the early symptoms of HIV disease are not serious and can easily be managed with good medical care. The progressive loss of CD4 cells and the spread of HIV in your body **is** serious. You may have HIV disease and not have any symptoms. As people take more and more responsibility for their recovery from addiction, they get many gifts. One major gift is a sense of self-empowerment about their total health care.

Persistent Low Grade Fever: Temperatures of 99 to 100 degrees F. that last for several days to several weeks, without other obvious causes like a cold or sinus infection.

Chronic Fatigue: Excessive tiredness after normal daily activities, such as climbing stairs, despite enough rest.

Swollen Lymph Glands: Unexpected appearance of multiple lumps in the neck, under the arms, or in the groin area that remain for several weeks.

Night Sweats: Sweats that usually occur without a fever. They often involve the whole body and may drench the bed linens.

Persistent Diarrhea: Lasts on and off of several weeks.

Unexplained Weight Loss: Loss of more than ten pounds, not as a result of dieting and despite eating a normal amount of food.

Skin Rashes: Itchy or scaly bumps or ulcers that appear anywhere on the body.

Lesions In The Mouth: Slow healing chancre sores or persistent white patches on the gums, tongue, or palate.

Genital Infections: Recurrent yeast infections in the vagina, or warts or ulcers on the penis, rectum, labia, or cervix.

Multiple Allergic Reactions: Increased severity of reactions (fever, rash, swelling, itching) to insect bites or common medications such as sulfa or penicillin.

This list is not to give you the information you need to self-diagnose. In sobriety, we neither self-diagnose nor self-medicate. Ignoring these symptoms would be massive denial, however. Let your doctor or other qualified medical people know about what is going on with you.

Knowledge about HIV and AIDS is particularly important to people who have alcoholism or other addictions because there are connections between the two diseases. What do you think are some of the connections? Brainstorm with the group and list the connections on the blackboard.

1. HIV can enter the body with IV needle use. People who use IV drugs are at high risk. The first disease, drug abuse or addiction can lead to a second, HIV disease.

2. Alcohol or other drugs can relax inhibitions. Alcohol and other drugs sometimes **lead to unsafe, promiscuous sexual behavior**. Have you ever had a sexual encounter that was unplanned, reckless, or in any way not a sober choice?

   Get High
   Get Stupid
   Get HIV

   Some drugs, like cocaine or speed, **can make people hyper-sexual**. Alcohol and other drugs **make people desperate** and desperate people do desperate things. Unsafe prostitution, having sex for money or drugs, is another connection.

3. Alcohol and other drug addiction make even the little things harder to do. Addiction often causes chaotic and impulsive lifestyles. Effective planning is much harder to do while using. Romance goes out the window. "What the Hell? Who cares? Why bother?"

4. Alcohol and other drugs **lower your resistance to HIV infection**. Using people get sick more easily than other people. Not everyone who comes into contact with HIV gets infected. If your CD4 cells are already suppressed, however, your body will not be as effective in rejecting HIV.

5. If you already have HIV, alcohol and other drugs may **stimulate HIV activation and replication**. This means they act as cofactors which suppress the immune system. Other cofactors include poor nutrition, negative mental attitudes, and other illnesses.

6. Drugs and alcohol **make mental health problems and neuropsychiatric problems associated with AIDS worse and more complicated**. It is impossible to really help people with mental health issues or a brain chemical imbalance when they are using. Is the depression caused by alcohol, the HIV, or a chemical imbalance? Most of us are aware of how alcohol can affect our thinking. HIV can also affect thinking.

7. Drugs and alcohol often **work against the medications associated with HIV management**. Therefore, a person who is already infected with HIV has a greater chance of getting sicker faster despite the best efforts of the medical team taking care of him/her.

There are also many similarities between HIV disease and addiction. Brainstorm with the group to develop an understanding of how these two diseases look alike.

1. Both carry **Stigma**. Many people with alcoholism, addiction, or HIV are ashamed. It is as if having a disease detracts from a person's character. This does not have to be.

2. Both carry **real or perceived prejudice**. Although it is unfortunate, there are many people in our society who look down on alcoholics/addicts and PWA's (people living with AIDS). Living in dignity and education are two ways to overcome other peoples' prejudice. How are you going to best confront this prejudice?

3. Both are marked by **alienation from families**. Has your addiction caused alienation in your family? Would or does HIV?

4. Both are **hidden diseases**. It is impossible to tell a person with HIV or an alcoholic in remission just by looking at them.

5. **Neither goes away.** *"Once you're a pickle, you'll never be a cucumber again!"* Once HIV is in the blood, it does not leave. You may never get sick with AIDS, but if you are infected, you have the capability of infecting others.

6. People living with either or both diseases sometimes characterize themselves by **"that's all I am."** While that can be a very real feeling, it simply is not true. Look around the room at your peers.

7. Both diseases can **carry a sense of "Why bother?"** Why bother getting sober? Why bother to take responsibility for HIV management? In an open question to the group, take some time to explore possible responses to these questions.

8. Both diseases fit Elizabeth Kubler-Ross's death and dying model.

   Denial
   Bargaining
   Anger
   Depression
   Acceptance

9. Both can be viewed as **Dis-Ease**. Disease is another way to describe inside pain. Both diseases carry more than their share. Sadness, despair, grief, anger, shame, guilt, frustration, hopelessness, and rage are just a few feelings associated with alcoholism and HIV.

10. Both can be viewed as **chronic** (lasting over time), **progressive** (getting worse), and **potentially fatal** (deadly) diseases.

Who Gets AIDS?

Currently, in this country, men who have had sex with other men and people who have shared needles are the largest groups of people infected with HIV. The numbers of women and teenagers infected with HIV are growing fast. This is **not** an issue of who you are or what labels you put on yourself. It is an issue of behavior.

What Behaviors?

The highest risk behaviors are receptive anal intercourse without a condom, and intravenous drug injection using shared equipment with other people. Unprotected vaginal intercourse is also risk behavior for both people. Brainstorm with the group as to other risk behaviors. ***There is no such thing as "safe sex." There is safer sex.*** Many behaviors will be your choice. It is important that they are choices and not just something you do.

HIV IS NOT A DEATH SENTENCE. Many people do not want to know if they carry HIV. They have a mindset, *"What I don't know won't hurt me,"* which is just not true. Responsible management of HIV can often keep people from getting sick. At the very least, early intervention can help people live longer and improve the quality of life.

To Test Or Not To Test

The question of testing is a highly personal one. For many of you, it may be too soon. Early recovery is a delicate time. Many of you are at a particularly emotionally vulnerable place. For others, testing now may be an appropriate action for your recovery. For all of you, making large life decisions by yourself is not recommended. *"We are not alone."* Who are some of the people you might talk to about taking the HIV test?

Sponsor
Husband/wife
Your doctor
A close sober friend
A counselor
A PWA

There are certain ground rules to consider before you decide to take an HIV test.

* Testing should only be done where there is both pre and post test individual counseling.

* Confidentiality of the results must be protected.

* You have a recovery program plan and a commitment to following through.

* You have an understanding of the people and agencies who help people with HIV. Where would you go with a positive test result?

* You have a clear understanding of what a negative test result means.

Open the group up to discussion and questions.

Close the group with a Confidentiality Circle.

To make it easier for you to access specific information including financial aid, we have included the key contacts for all 50 states, the District of Columbia, Puerto Rico, and the Virgin Islands.

Please copy your appropriate Health Dept. and attach it to the end of the client Handout, along with other local resources they can use when they leave treatment.

STATE HEALTH DEPARTMENTS HIV RESOURCES

Alaska Dept of Health
Office of Epidemiology
Division of Public Health
3601 C Street, Suite 540
Anchorage, AK 99524
907/561-4406

Alabama Dept of Public Health
AIDS/STD Program
434 Monroe Street
Montgomery, AL 36130
205/242-5609

Arkansas Dept of Health
AIDS/STD Program
4815 West Markham, Slot 33
Little Rock, AR 72205
501/661-2135

Arizona Dept of Health
Division Of Disease Prevention
30018 N 3rd St, Room 203
Phoenix, AZ 85012
601/230-5819

California Dept of Health Services
Office of AIDS
830 S Street, Box 942732
Sacramento, CA 94234
916/445-0553

Colorado Dept of Health
STD/AIDS Education/Risk Reduction
4210 E 11th Ave
Denver, CO 80220
303/692-2680

Connecticut Dept of Health Services
AIDS Program
150 Washington Street
Hartford, CT 06106
203/566-1157

DC Commission on Public Health
AIDS Program
1660 L Street, NW, Suite 700
Washington, DC 20036
202/673-3679

Delaware Dept of Health and Social Services
AIDS Program Office
3000 Newport Gap Pike, Bldg G
Wilmington, DE 19808
302/995-8422

Florida Dept Health/Rehabilitation Services
Health Education and Risk Reduction
1317 Winewood Blvd, Bldg 2
Tallahassee, FL 32399
904/487-2478

Georgia Dept of Human Resources
Communicable Disease Branch
HIV/AIDS Ryan White Project
878 Peachtree St NE, Room 109
Atlanta, GA 30309
404/894-5122

Hawaii Dept of Health
STD/AIDS Prevention Branch
3627 Kilauea Ave, Suite 306
Honolulu, HI 96816
808/735-5303

Iowa Dept of Public Health
AIDS Prevention Program
Lucas State Office Bldg, 1st floor
515/281-4938

Idaho Dept of Health and Welfare
AIDS Program
Communicable Disease Prevention Bureau
450 W State Street
Boise, ID 83720
208/334-5930

Illinois Dept of Public Health
AIDS Activity
160 N LaSalle St, 7th Floor S
Chicago, IL 60601
312/814-4846

Indiana State Board of Health
Division of Acquired Disease
Box 1964, Room 232
Indianapolis, IN 46206
317/633-0851

Kansas Dept of Health and Environment
AIDS Program
Mills Building, Suite 605
109 SW 9th Street
Topeka, KS 66612
913/296-0022

Kentucky Dept for Health Services
AIDS Education
275 E Main Street
Frankfort, KY 40621
502/564-6539

Louisiana Dept of Health and Environment
STD Section
Box 60630
New Orleans, LA 70160
504/568-5275

Massachusetts Dept of Public Health
AIDS Bureau
150 Tremont Street, 11th Floor
Boston, MA 02111
617/727-0368

Maryland Dept of Health and Mental Hygiene
AIDS Administration
201 w Preston Street
Baltimore, MD 21201
301/225-5019

Maine Bureau of Health
Office of AIDS
State House, Station 11
Augusta, ME 04333
207/287-3747

Michigan Dept of Health
HIV/AIDS Prevention
3423 N Logan, Box 30195
Lansing, MI 48909
517/335-8371

Minnesota Dept of Health
AIDS/STD Prevention Services
717 SE Delaware Street
Minneapolis, MN 55440
612/623-5698

Missouri Dept of Health
bureau of AIDS Prevention
Box 570
Jefferson City, MO 65102
314/751-6438

Mississippi Dept of Health
HIV/AIDS Prevention Program
Box 1700
Jackson, MS 39215
601/9607723

Montana Dept of Health
AIDS Program
Cogswell Bldg
Helena, MT 59620
406/444-3565

North Carolina Health Dept
HIV/STD Control Branch
Box 27687
Raleigh, NC 27611
919/733-7301

North Dakota Dept of Health
AIDS Project
State Capitol Bldg
600 E Blvd
Bismark, ND 58505
701/224-2370

Nebraska Dept of Health
AIDS Program/Disease Control
Box 95007
301 Centennial Mall
Lincoln, NE 68509
402/471-2937

New Hampshire Dept of Health and Welfare
STD/HIV Program
6 Hazen Drive
Concord, NH 03301
603/271-4576

New Jersey Dept of Health
Division on AIDS Prevention and Control
CN 360, 363 W State Street
Trenton, NJ 08625
609/984-6000

New Mexico Dept of Health
AIDS Prevention Program
1190 St Francis Drive
Santa Fe, NM 87502
505/827-0086

Nevada State Health Division
Bureau of Disease Control
505 E King Street
Room 304
Carson City, NV 89710
702/687-4800

New York State Dept of Health
AIDS Drug Assistance Program
14 Computer Dr West
Albany, NY 12205
518/459-1641

Ohio Dept of Health
AIDS Activity Unit
Box 118
Columbus, OH 43266
614/466-5480

Oklahoma Dept of Health
STD/AIDS Division
1000 NE Tenth Street
Oklahoma City, OK 73152
405/271-4636

Oregon Dept of Health
AIDS Program
800 NE Oregon, Suite 745
Portland, OR 97232
503/731-4029

Pennsylvania Dept of Health
Bureau of HIV/AIDS
Box 90/Room 913
Harrisburg, PA 17120
717/783-0479

Commonwealth of Puerto Rico Dept of Health
STD Control Program
Box 71423
San Juan, PR 00936
809/754-8118

Rhode Island Dept of Health
AIDS/STD Division
3 Capitol Hill
Room 105
Providence, RI 02908
401/277-2320

South Carolina Dept of Health
HIV/AIDS Division
Box 101106
Michael Jarrett Bldg
Columbia, SC 29211
803/734-5482

South Dakota Dept of Health
AIDS Program
523 E Capital
Pierre, SD 57501
605/773-3357

Tennessee Dept of Health
AIDS Program
C 2-221 Cordell Hull Bldg
Nashville, TN 37219
615/741-7500

Texas Dept of Health
HIV Division
1100 W 49th Street
Austin, TX 78756
512/458-7209

Utah Dept of Health
Bureau of HIV/AIDS
288 North, 1460 West, Box 16660
Salt Lake City, UT 84116
801/538-6096

Virginia Dept of Health
AIDS Activity Program
Box 2448/Room #112
Richmond, VA 23218
804/225-4844

Virgin Islands Dept of Health
AIDS Program
Charles Harwood Complex
Christiansted, VI 00820
809/776-8311

Virgin Islands Dept of Health
AIDS Program
48 Sugar Estate
St Thomas, VI 00802
809/776-3168 (St Croix)

Vermont Dept of Health
HIV/AIDS Education Program
60 Main Street, Box 70
Burlington, VT 05402
802/863-7245

Washington State Dept of Health
Division of HIV/AIDS & STD's
PO Box 47844
Olympia, WA 98504
206/586-8344

Wisconsin Dept of Health and Social Services
AIDS/HIV Program
1414 E Washington Ave/Rm 241
Madison, WI 53703
608/267-5287

West Virginia Dept of Health
AIDS Education Program
1422 Washington Street E
Charleston, WV 25301
304/558-5358

Wyoming Division of Health and Medical Services
Preventive Medicine/AIDS Program
Hathaway Bldg, 4th Floor
Cheyenne, WY 82002
307/777-7953

INTRODUCTION TO THE STEPS

Notes to Clinicians:

These are suggested guidelines to correspond to the way we have presented the Steps.

There are two levels to the steps. At one level we want our client to understand intellectually and emotionally their powerlessness and the consequences of their addiction. Initially, the client needs to identify the problem, their addiction, and their unmanageability in order to achieve freedom. They do this by **"working the Steps".**

At another level, the *meta-level,* the clients are actually entering a spiritual path. In the spiritual path, the Hero needs to slay the dragon to experience enlightenment. To do this, the Hero needs new weapons and guides. **These *are* the Steps.**

The challenge to the clinician is to present both levels of the Steps because both levels exist.

Initially, we ask the client to work at a superficial level, level one, listing the facts about their addiction. After a few pages we drop the client from their head to their emotions, their deeper awareness of feelings. Eventually, we connect them to a spiritual awareness, their greater selves.

We have provided directions throughout the Step Workbooks to do this. We have directed the client to initially keep the answers short and simple. A few pages later we direct them to attach a feeling to their responses. Then we ask them to assign meaning to their lives.

Before handing out the Step Workbooks, assign the appropriate preliminary readings. For example, *"Before you start Step One, you need to read the AA "Big Book", Chapter 5, then read Step 1 in the "Twelve Steps And Twelve Traditions". "Come back in two days and I'll give you the Step One Workbook."* For Narcotics Anonymous, assign Chapters 3 and 4 and Step 1 in the NA Basic Text.

There are also directions in the Workbooks for the client to complete only a few pages and before progressing, to check it out with their counselor. This gives you the opportunity to help focus the client and keep them on track.

We also suggest reviewing the directions in a small group. This gives clients the benefit of hearing each other's questions, and you the opportunity to clarify, clarify, clarify, expectations.

Step One is Handout #13.
Step Two is Handout #14.
Step Three is Handout #15.

STEP 1

Step 1: We admitted we were powerless over alcohol - that our lives had become unmanageable.

The same way that alcohol affects every cell in our body, the disease of alcoholism or chemical dependency affects every aspect of our lives. In the beginning, this is hard for us to accept. It's called denial and every person who has wanted to recover from chemical dependency had to look at and work through their denial. Step 1 is often the most difficult part of our recovery because our denial is so strong. Our denial has protected us from **feeling** the consequences of our disease, namely, how our disease has lied to us and hurt those we love.

If you are reading this, be aware that this was an action **you are** taking. You have a choice to put this down now and walk away. There is no gun to your head. No matter what the circumstances are which lead you to treatment, you can always refuse to do this Step 1. If you have been coerced into treatment by your boss, family, or doctor, the reality is that you can quit your job, get a divorce, and change doctors. We always have a choice about doing Step 1.

Listen to our stories in AA, NA, and CA. None of us wanted to look at the reality of our addiction. We have all been in each other's shoes whether we are angry, resistant, afraid, or confused. Listen to our stories. Each of us who is recovering will somehow relate to you a gift of our humanity, that somehow we found a place within ourselves that could be honest, which could be open, and was willing. If you are reading this, you are already open and willing.

Your honesty will bring you pain. The psychologist, Carl Jung, tells us that "There is no birth of consciousness without pain." We can keep our denial and stay exactly the way we are, or we can put our denial aside, feel the pain of the disease our denial protects us from, and become conscious, awake, and alive. When the lie of our denial is aside, we can begin to discover who we truly are. In freeing ourselves from the bonds of our disease, we give birth to the human within it.

We are like chicks struggling to emerge from our egg shell. If our mothers have to break the shell, we die. Only we can peck through our shell to the warmth of the sun and the freedom beyond it. Like the chick who will die if their shell is only partly open, this freedom requires the willingness to peck away one section at a time, but the shell must be slowly and **completely** removed.

Make a decision about doing this Step 1. Walk away if you already know that you cannot be honest or open to looking at your disease. Should you decide to do this, expect the unexpected. You are about to begin the adventure into a life that is second to none.

You are about to begin a journey into the unknown. As with all journeys, mythical or real, you will need to take special tools or weapons with you to slay the dragon, to open secret gates, and to give you courage and strength. Prepare for your journey and gather your tools.

The Step 1 journey is about discovering truth. It's about discovering powerlessness and unmanageability over alcohol or other chemicals. The tools you will need are found in The Big Book of AA, in How It Works, Chapter 5. Before starting this Step, slowly read every word of the first few pages. It is filled with the directions about the tools you will need around honesty, open-mindedness, and willingness.

This is the first direction: Read How It Works.

During the rest of this workbook, take one question at a time.
Keep your answers **simple** and under five sentence responses at most.

This is the second direction: Do a page or two and check it out with your counselors.

SECTION I: POWERLESSNESS

The disease of alcoholism or chemical dependency is **chronic, progressive,** and **incurable.** This section deals with looking at those areas.

In the chart below, simply look at the facts around your use. If you need more space, make another chart on a larger piece of paper, or tape the continuation of the chart to this sheet. Draw a horizontal line across the chart to indicate a change in using or using pattern. If you need help,there is a sample chart on the following page.

USING HISTORY CHART

Age	Type of Chemical	Amount	How Often	For How Long
First Use				

Sample:

Please note in the sample, that when the person's using changed, whether it was the amount used, the type of chemical, the frequency, or times of day, the person started another column. If you have only used alcohol, include looking at the different types of alcohol. If there were times that you were completely abstinent from all mind altering chemicals, make a note of those years with an explanation. Most of us think that our using was pretty much the same from year to year, doing this helps us see our denial.

Age	Type of Chemical	Amount	How Often	For How Long
12	beer	3 beers	Fri. & Sat. nights 8pm-12pm	4 years
16	beer	6 beers	Fri. & Sat. nights 8pm-12pm	1 year
16	marijuana	1 joint	Fri. & Sat.	1 year
17	beer	6 beers	Thurs. thru Sun. nights 8pm-2am	2 years
	marijuana	2 joints	Daily	2 years
	speed, etc.	5 hits "white cross"	4 days a week	6 months

CHRONIC:

Chronic means that you've had the disease a long time.

Looking back at your chart, what is the total # of years that you've used each chemical? List them below:

What is the total # of years that you've been using?

PROGRESSIVE:

Progression means that our using becomes worse. This is seen in two ways:

1. We increase our **tolerance** to the chemical, or can use more.

2. The **frequency** of our using increases, we use more often or for longer periods of time.

When did your tolerance change?

How did your tolerance change?

Looking back on this, at what age do you see yourself crossing the line from normal using?

Looking back at your chart, are you only addicted to a single chemical? List it below.

Are you or have you been poly addicted or cross addicted? List the chemicals below. Circle your **favorite** drug or drug combinations. This is your drug of choice.

The drug used the most often is also the drug of choice. Which is it?

There are other physical symptoms of chemical dependency. **Blackouts** or periods of amnesia, is a major sign that somebody is alcoholic. Two or more blackouts indicate a sure sign of alcoholism.

List Blackouts that you have had. Start with the first one, the last one, and one in the middle. Include your age, how much you were using, how long the blackout lasted, and how you knew that you'd had one afterwards.

1.

2.

3.

This is the third direction: For the rest of Step 1, if the question has a * next to it, the question wants you to include in your answer:

your age
the type and amount of the chemical used
the circumstances

LOSS OF CONTROL:

Loss of control is another symptom of chemical dependency. While there are many aspects of loss of control, in this section we will look at the loss of control over the actual use.

* List times you said you were not going to drink or use and still did.

1.

2.

3.

* List times you used more than you intended to.

1.

2.

3.

The condition **"stupor"** occurs when the brain is so intoxicated that it begins to lose neurological function. Stupor is characterized by slurred speech, lack of coordination, and an unsteady walk.

* List times that you have been neurologically impaired and in a stupor.

1.

2.

3.

Passing out is a drug overdose. The brain is so impaired that it loses its ability to function. The medical term for a pass out is **coma.** The individual stays in the coma until their body can eliminate the poisons from their brain.

* List times that you have been in a coma.

1.

2.

3.

Looking back now, at what age did your disease begin to show?

LOSS OF CONTROL:

Attempts to control use:

A classic symptom of middle stage chemical dependence is the attempt to control use. *This is not about trying to quit, but to control the using.* This may be done consciously or unconsciously. An **unconscious** example is that of the person who switches from hard alcohol to beer, feeling that the liquor has some kind of negative effect. They're *not trying to quit,* just trying to control the strong effects of the alcohol. A **conscious** example is when you"ve decided to make rules about your using. Some examples of this are changing the type, frequency, and amount of the chemical used, like *"I'll only drink on weekends"* or *"I'll only smoke pot."*

* List **unconscious** examples of attempts to control your use.

1.

2.

* List three ways that you tried to **consciously** control your use and why.

1.

2.

3.

Go back to the above five answers in "Attempts to control use" . Add to those answers in the spaces below by including : **Did it work? What happened at a feeling level so you lost control again?**
For example: If my rule was to only drink on weekends (when I was 30-years old), my response below to that answer would be: "It only worked for **three weeks.** I was **feeling lonely** during the week and started going out and drinking with my friends again."

Complete all the answers to those questions in the spaces below.

1.

2.

3.

4.

5.

So, looking at your new answers, what **feelings** are you the most likely to use over?

1.

2.

3.

Serious attempts to control using are **attempts to quit.** In the space below, add examples of your attempts to quit. Include factors such as your age, the type of drug, the reason why, how long it lasted, the circumstance, and feelings you started using over again.

1.

2.

3.

Again, list your using **feelings:**

1.

2.

3.

Which are the two main feelings which will cause relapse for you?

1.

2.

How can you handle them in sobriety?

1.

2.

To sum up this section, chemical dependence is a disease that is **chronic, progressive, incurable,** and characterized by **increasing tolerance** and **loss of control**. Write a sentence or two to prove that you have the disease.

Go back over the work you've done.
What surprised you?

What did you see differently about your disease?

What was the hardest part for you to answer?

The hardest part tells you about where you still have denial. Where do you still have denial about your using?

How do you see that you are powerless over chemicals?

How do you see that you are powerless over your disease?

SECTION II: UNMANAGEABILITY

Unmanageability has many meanings. Generally, it means that you have had **consequences as a result of your using.** Powerlessness means that despite the consequences, you've kept on using. Seeing and accepting powerlessness is the easy part. ***Seeing and accepting unmanageability in every area of your life is your next challenge.*** Our monster denial is usually very skilled at keeping us from the truth.

Most of us can see our unmanageability in some areas - *"Yes my drinking affected my health but not my children"* or vice versa. *If your drinking did not affect your children, why quit drinking? They love you when you're drunk!* ***For you to quit using, leave no stone unturned.*** Those stones are your denial and every stone which remains gives you permission to drink or use again - *"It wasn't that bad, it didn't bother my kids. Pour me another. "*

While unmanageability affects every area of our lives, these are the main areas we will be exploring: Physical, emotional, spiritual, intellectual, financial, sexual, social and familial. Remember that your denial has protected you from **feeling** your disease. As you **confront** your denial, these feelings will surface. The gifts they will give you are innumerable: The truth of your disease, the pain of your disease, compassion for yourself and others, sadness, and loss. These are some of the precious parts of our humanity that we have lost or numbed in our need to keep using. These are feelings which create our depth and are parts of our spirit.

The directions are simple and are to be followed throughout the rest of the Step where appropriate.

This is the fourth direction: To be able to see the chronicity and progression of the unmanageability, continue to include your age, what and how much you were using. In addition to your explanation, add the feeling that you now have as you answer the questions.

PHYSICAL CONSEQUENCES:

* List all the ways your body has been affected by which drug. (Include physical problems, permanent or temporary, include throwing up).

1.

2.

3.

4.

5.

* List the ways your brain has been affected. (Include memory, seizures, concentration, headaches, hangovers, etc.).

1.

2.

3.

When our brain is impaired, we are at high risk for accidents.
* List accidents that you've had and how your were hurt.

1.

2.

3.

* How have you experienced withdrawal? To which drugs?

1.

2.

3.

4.

Which chemical was hardest on your body? Explain.

At what **age** did your body begin to show the effects? Explain.

How many more years did you use?

What do **others** think are the worst physical consequences?

What do **you** think is the worst physical consequence?

Where have you had the most denial?

EMOTIONAL CONSEQUENCES:

Prolonged use of chemicals affects our brain. Emotions are partly based on brain and body chemistry. Altering these body chemicals affects our ability to feel normal. List ways your emotional health has changed. (Include depression, irritability, mood swings, outbursts, anxiety, etc.).

1.

2.

3.

Because of our denial, we blame problems on other things, not our drinking. What types of problems did you develop and try to solve without quitting using, how did you try to solve them, did it work, what happened?

1.

2.

3.

Did you ever see a therapist? Did you talk about your using? What happened?

1.

2.

What do others see as your largest area of emotional unmanageability? Be specific.

What do you see?

Where is your denial here?

SPIRITUAL UNMANAGEABILITY:

Spiritual health is a huge concept. It relates to our ability to feel at peace with ourselves and others. It's about who we are in our hearts. Our sense of purpose, of belonging, of giving and sacrifice, creativity, capacity to give and receive love, joy and pain are all aspects of being a spiritual person. Our using deeply wounds us spiritually and we become people we don't recognize or know anymore.

List the ways your disease has affected you spiritually:

How has it affected your sense of purpose?

Feelings of serenity and peace?

Ability to be accepting?

Ability to give love?

To receive love?

Your dignity and self respect?

Your creativity?

When we lose our spirituality, we become self-centered. We get what we want or need instead of working things out, compromising or holding back. For some of us, our self-centeredness is subtle: We spend time drinking instead of being with our kids, or we'll buy drugs or things for ourselves instead of something our spouse or friend may need. For others of us, our self-centeredness is not so subtle: We lie, cheat, steal, or become violent to get our way. **It's all the same, without our spirit, all forms of self-centeredness keeps us spiritually wounded.** To continue to use, we act in ways which wound our spirits. How have you become self-centered?
Remember to include all of the responses in Direction # 4.

Lies I have told under the influence:

1.

2.

Lies I have told about my using:

1.

2.

Ways I have cheated:

1.

2.

Things I have stolen:

1.

2.

Unkind things I have done:

1.

2.

How I have embarrassed others:

1.

2.

Violence or acts of violence:

1.

2.

Ways I have been uncaring:

1.

2.

Promises I have broken:

1.

2.

Who are you when you are using?

Is this who you really are?

Has your spiritual life become unmanageable?

What has been your greatest spiritual loss?

Who can you be if you stay clean and sober?

EFFECTS ON FAMILY:

Our families and relationships are **always** affected by our disease. **This is usually the most painful part to acknowledge.** In our hearts, we love them, we try to protect them, we would rather die than hurt them. Our disease takes this away from us, our denial keeps us from seeing it. We hurt those we love, who love us.

List your family members below. How has your disease harmed them? Give a **specific** example. A vague example like, "I have lied to my wife", is meaningless. For you to see your disease, you need to give specific examples like, "I lied to my wife last week. I told her I lost the money, but I really spent it on a fifth of vodka." You may use the same person more than once. Fill the page:

Family Member	Hurtful Behavior	Example
1.		
2.		
3.		
4.		
5.		
6.		
7.		
8.		
9.		
10.		

Would you do these things normally?

Are you powerless?

Where has been your biggest area of denial?

SEXUAL UNMANAGEABILITY:

Chemicals and addiction affect our sexuality. Some of us become more promiscuous, others more isolated. We may become more selfish and demanding, or disinterested and withholding. We may be inappropriate. 70 to 80% of male alcoholics experience impotence, some of us become more violent. List ways your sexuality has been affected. Be specific:

1.

2.

3.

Where is your biggest area of denial?

INTELLECTUAL UNMANAGEABILITY:

Most of us like to think we are intellectual giants. Some of us believe we are more stupid than gnats. Eventually, we figure out that both beliefs are a result of distorted thinking. In this section, we will be looking at some reality. The chemicals themselves and our love affair with our addiction results in intellectual unmanageability. Chemicals affect our brain, our memories, our ability to problem solve and abstract. The addictive lifestyle affects our ability to grow and develop intellectually. We stop learning things because we are preoccupied with using.

How have chemicals affected your ability to problem solve? Be specific:

1.

2.

How have you become intellectually stunted? (Look at level of education, interests, and hobbies abandoned. Do you watch television versus reading, is your level of conversation with people superficial? What types of people you interact with?

1.

2.

3.

4.

Was this your plan for the future?

Is this unmanageable?

Where is your biggest area of denial?

SOCIAL UNMANAGEABILITY:

This is another difficult section to examine, primarily for two reasons. First our using has been so chronic (or long) that the changes in our social life are subtle at first. Secondly, like looking at our families, this can be painful. With this section, again look at your age, the circumstances, and write a line or two telling about the story to be specific. If you cannot answer all of the questions, your denial is very strong.

When our disease progresses, we have to change friends who use more like we do. Which straight friends did you drop or spend less time with? Explain.

1.

2.

3.

Who dropped you because of your using? How do you know? Explain.

1.

2.

3.

Which friendship did you develop so that you could use with them? Explain.

Which friends have you lied to and betrayed?

1.

2.

3.

What have you done to your friends that you regret?

1.

2.

3.

4.

5.

Which of your friends need to know that you cannot drink or use anymore?

1.

2.

3.

4.

Which people do you need to end relationships with?

1.

2.

3.

How and when will you do this?

1.

2.

3.

Where do you still have denial about your social unmanageability?

FINANCIAL UNMANAGEABILITY

Our chemical dependency has cost us thousands, thousands, and thousands of dollars, directly and indirectly.

The **direct cost** is what it has cost us directly out of pocket. Go back through your using history and add up the cost you paid **for each drink or drug. Go all the way back and add year by year.** *Use a separate page to show your figures.*

What is the total amount that you have spent on chemicals?

A. ____________

Our friends, family, dealer, bartender, etc., give us our chemicals. Sometimes we steal them. Add up the total cost your chemicals would have cost had you paid for them. What is the total cost your chemicals cost others?

B.____________

Add A & B. What is the total cost of your direct chemical use?

C.____________

Our addictions have cost us and others **indirectly**. These are secondary costs. They include medical bills, increased insurance, accidents, court costs, loss of work,or paying alimony, child support, jail time, car wrecks, lost items, bad deals, court fines. **Add up the up the secondary costs you have paid or monies you could have earned.** Include medical bills, insurance, lost wages, court fines, etc. If you dropped out of school or never went but intended to, add up your lost salary through the years.

What is the total cost **to you?** **D.** ____________

Our chemical dependency **cost other people money.** What we cannot do or pay falls on society's shoulders. Sick leave costs our companies. Unemployment, welfare, social services, prison, unpaid medical bills and landlords, accidents to others, delinquent debts and bills, etc., are all burdens we have placed on others because of our disease and under responsibility. How much have you cost society?

E.____________

Add D & E. What is your total cost to yourself, your family, and society?

F. ____________

Add C & F. What is the total and complete cost of your addiction?

G. ____________

What do you **think** about this?

How do you **feel** about this?

Have you experienced financial unmanageability?

Where is your denial still strong around your finances?

SUMMARY

Now that you have finished this workbook, go back through the pages and review it. Add things you have remembered, be more honest in other places. Our recovery depends upon our ability to be brutally honest.

What are some of the feelings you have experienced in doing this work?

How will they be gifts to you in your recovery?

In a few sentences below, pretend you need to explain to a newcomer that you are chemically dependent. How would you tell them that you have admitted that you are powerless over your addiction and that your life has become unmanageable?

If you have completed every answer, what have you learned about yourself by being able to do this?

What parts of your spirit have you reclaimed on this part of your journey through the Steps?

When you do this work, when you allow yourself to have your feelings, when you share this story with others, be aware that you are now in recovery. It is the first step.

May you feel the dignity of being an honest person again. This is the spiritual principle of the first Step, that peace comes through honesty. Go in peace and may you feel blessed.

STEP TWO

Step 2: Came to believe that a power greater than ourselves could restore us to sanity.

In Step 1, we learned that we have a disease which is chronic, progressive and fatal. We saw through our years of experience that there was nothing we could do to control it or change it. So now what?

Step 2 tells us that we came to believe that a power greater than ourselves could restore us to sanity. This step tells us many things. It tells us that a power greater than ourselves, not our egos, not our self will, not our plans or determination will restore us to sanity: **A power greater than ourselves.** It informs us that to recover, **we** aren't going to fix the problem, not by ourselves. Our brain and thoughts deceived us in the first place. In AA, they tell us that "My best thinking got me here."

Our brain can only tell us what we already know. It can't give us new information or a better way to deal with the same problem it's been struggling with already. **This is important to accept.** Many alcoholics fall by the wayside because once sober, they think they magically know all the solutions.

Imagine a person who's been diagnosed with cancer saying, *"Thanks for telling me I have cancer, I think I'll leave now. I can figure out a way to cure it."* This is part of the insanity mentioned in the second part of the Step. We are simply people like others with a chronic disease who realize that we don't know how to treat it. When diagnosed with cancer, most people then ask, *"What can I do about it?"* Since they don't know, they are asking the experts, **a power greater than themselves.** To recover from addiction, we do the same thing.

The word sanity is derived from the Latin word "sanus". Sanus means "healthy." In other words, Step 2 informs us that as with other diseases, to recover, we need to believe that something greater than ourselves can restore us to health.

Another way to look at the idea of sanity is to understand it as meaning mental health. Step 2 implies that when we are drinking and using we are mentally unhealthy, or insane. For some of us, this may be a hard pill to swallow. We will be tempted to exclaim, *"I'm not insane! I don't need a psychiatrist!"* There are two facts which contradict us. First, normal people don't do what we do to get our chemicals. To them this is crazy. Secondly, it is incomprehensible to imagine living the lives of pain and degradation which we endure. To continue drinking and using knowing now the horrendous consequences we suffer, **is insane.** In Step 2, we believe we can be restored to sanity. Like the person with cancer, it requires finding a power greater than ourselves who can help us with our disease.

Part I - Our Insanity

Our denial keeps us from seeing ourselves the way the rest of the world sees us. It is difficult to accept that we have been irrational, insane. We are out of step with the rest of the world. To recover, we *first* need to see the insanity of our using and using behaviors. How else could we convince ourselves to quit using unless we were convinced that our using is crazy?

Give examples of situations you were in while intoxicated that would be considered insane (include your age and how you feel about it today).

1.

2.

3.

How did you distort reality to explain these situations to yourself and others to appear "normal"?

1.

2.

3.

Give examples of times people tried to tell you that you needed to change and why (include your age and how you feel about it today). Were they correct?

1.

2.

3.

How did you avoid making the changes?

1.

2.

3.

Give examples of things you can't believe have happened in your life as a result of your addiction. Do normal people try to do this to themselves?

1.

2.

3.

How do you think others see you as a result of this behavior?

How do you see your using behavior?

Part II - Powers Greater Than Ourselves

A power greater than ourselves is something which helps us recover from our addiction. This "power" is something which understands our addiction and can show us how to recover. It is usually some form of Teacher or Guide from whom we can obtain direction and with whom we can have contact. We find these powers outside of ourselves because we have already seen that we don't have the answers. If we did, we wouldn't be powerless.

Here's a story showing us an example of how many of us lived before recovery and before doing this Step:

Early in spring, there was a great rain. Newly sober, Joe watched as the water rose. He felt convinced that his trust and faith in his new found "Higher Power" would protect and save him. The National Guard came by when the water was up to the foundation of his house, calling him to join them and evacuate the area.

"No," said Joe. "I believe I will be saved and protected." The guardsmen left when they realized their efforts to save the man were futile. The water continued rising and now engulfed the first floor of Joe's home. On the now-raging river outside, a boatman stopped, offering Joe a way to safety. "No", said Joe. "I will survive this flood. I have a Higher Power which will save me".

When the flood water reached the second floor, Joe perched himself on the roof, still convinced of his survival. A helicopter landed besided him on the roof. "Come, hurry, you cannot possibly live through this," the pilot urged. Again, Joe refused to be saved.

Within a half hour, Joe found himself engulfed by the water, unprepared and drowning. To his Higher Power he screamed, "How could you let this happen? I depended on you to save me!"

A voice spoke, "I came to save you three times and you refused my help."

The End

Even those of us with enormous, unshakable faith in God as our Higher Power, find that in addition to our faith, there are additional powers greater than our thinking to help us with our disease.

For those of us who are atheists, this Step does not tell us to get "religious". **For all of us,** it says, believe that there is something greater than you which can help. Come to believe this.

Step Two

List some powers greater than you which can save you from the destruction of your disease. Powers which can restore you to sanity, or health. Give examples of how they are useful:

1.

2.

3.

4.

5.

6.

7.

8.

9.

10.

The spiritual gift in Step 2 is the gift of openness. A great Master, or a person living their spirituality, is a person who fully recognizes that they are always a student. One of the wonderful aspects of being in recovery is that we are given a gift of exploring other's paths, new ways to live and grow. We are given full permission to discard old ideas we thought were facts of life. Old ideas which kept us sick and shut off from the world and others. We are finally given the freedom to be imperfect and to look outside in the world for new solutions. We are allowed to be who we are, ongoing students in our ongoing life.

A symptom of being back in our disease is when we believe that we have all the answers. When we believe that we don't need any help or suggestions because we know the best solutions. A person in their disease is somebody who is "closed off" to the powers greater than themselves. A person in recovery is open to their spirit, to new directions on their path.

How will you know if you are in your disease?

1.

2.

3.

What commitment will you make if this happens?

1.

2.

3.

What situations or problems in sobriety do you already have answers for?

1.

2.

3.

To stay open to your new teachers and guides, what will you do when you are being closed minded, opinionated or resistant?

1.

2.

3.

Step 1 show us that we are powerless over our addiction and that our lives are unmanageable. Step 1 provides us with honesty and humility.

Step 2 gives us hope that we can recover, **but only if we look outside of ourselves for the solutions.** Step 2 transforms us spiritually by allowing us to become hopeful and open. Step 2 leads us to Step 3. When you believe you have found some powers greater than yourself, you are ready for the next step in your journey — Step 3, reaping the benefits and teachings of these new powers.

STEP THREE

Step 3 : Made a decision to turn our will and our lives over to the care of God, as we understood Him.

Many of us gasp, *"Not God! I'm not ready to become religious!"* Luckily for you, nobody says you have to. Upon examination of this Step you will notice it reads "God, as we understand Him." Whatever you listed as powers greater than yourself in Step 2 fits the bill exactly for Step 3. There are many parts to this Step. The first part of the Step says that we "made a decision." Since we work our program one day at a time, this Step asks that **we make a decision just for today.**

The second part of this Step says that we turn our will and our lives over. *"Our will"* means our thoughts and beliefs. For example, a person who is "strong willed" is a person who is stubborn or opinionated. *"Our lives"* means our actions and behaviors.

"God as we understand Him" means the power which we have come to believe will restore us to sanity. Some of us call this power our Higher Power. If some of you have AA as a Higher Power, then this is what you will turn your thinking and actions over to.

This is a very simple Step. It suggests that to recover, we decide that just for today, **no matter what,** we give our thinking and actions over to that Higher Power. In other words, *we don't give ourselves directions, we follow directions from another source.*

In Step 2 we become open. **In Step 3 we are teachable and follow our new guides.**

Some of us already have an understanding of God or a Higher Power before we get sober. For those of us who don't, we use a simple formula to help us follow directions. God may mean, <u>G</u>ood, <u>O</u>rderly, <u>D</u>irection. Is what we are doing in our recovery:

<u>G</u>ood for our recovery?

Providing <u>O</u>rder in our lives?

Giving us <u>D</u>irection towards sobriety?

The spiritual principle in Step 3 is about willingness. *"How it Works"* in the Big Book of Alcoholics Anonymous tells us that to recover, we need to be willing to go to any length. It outlines the need to avoid half measures. Step 3 puts our willingness into action.

What is *God as you understand Him?*

What are the Higher Powers you will turn your will and your life over to?

1.

2.

3.

How do you recognize a Higher Power's help?

What will you do if you disagree with the directions?

How do you plan to make decisions to stay sober and follow directions today?

1.

2.

3.

Steps 1, 2 and 3 lay the foundation for the rest of our recovery which is outlined in the remaining Steps. **We don't stop at Step 3.** *A house with just the foundation is still not a house, we can't live in it.*

The rest of the Steps show us how to build our lives, how to create rooms and spaces within ourselves we never believed possible. It is a wonderful journey and we pray that you travel to the end to join us.

By completing and sharing these first three Steps you have already begun to change.

What is different about you today?

CHECK IN

This group can be very useful in helping clients begin to clarify feelings and increase awareness of their physical, emotional, and spiritual condition at the beginning of each treatment day. It identifies feelings and separates issues. "Check in" directs clients to formulate goals in the recovery process on a daily basis, reinforcing the idea of "one day at a time" by teaching them how to set realistic goals and to follow through with action. In addition, it also provides staff with crucial information about each client and helps take the pulse of the group for the day.

This is not a process group. The benefit is in its simplicity and the staff's ability to redirect in a supportive, non-threatening manner. "Keep it simple".

Ask the group sit in a circle.

Directions to the group:

"We will be going around the room giving each person a chance to check in on a physical, emotional, and spiritual level. We will also ask you to set a goal for the day. If you are new, we will help you with the format."

1. **Physical Check in:** *"The physical check in pertains to how your body is feeling right now, as you sit in group. Be specific about it . Do you have aches and pains? Where? Do you have high or low energy?"*

Note:
Addicts, by history, are usually out of touch with their bodies. This part of their check in allows them to begin to notice and respond to their body's messages.

In the physical check-in, clients need to describe how their bodies feel.
Example: *"Physically, I feel well-rested, I have tension in my shoulders and neck. I feel hungry."*

2. **Emotional Check in:** *"Being clear about our feelings and understanding the difference between a thought and feeling is important for all of us."* Some basic helpful hints include:

   Avoid the words: Good, fine, bad, or other vague words like wonderful or terrific. The point is to define your feelings so that other members of the group have a **clear idea** of what your **feelings** are. If you are not clear we will ask you to be more specific. You can use the feeling list to help you.

Note:
Explain that all feelings can be boiled down into these core feelings:

Sad (Pain)	Love
Mad (Anger)	Happy
Bad (Shame/Guilt)	Peaceful
Fear	Hopeful
Helpless	Harmonious
Alone/Empty	

It's helpful to have these core feelings posted nearby on the group room wall. If a client checks in with, *"I feel irritated today,"* point to the list and ask him to be more specific. "Irritated" is a cover-up feeling for low-grade **anger**. There are solutions for anger. Clarifying "irritated" allows the client the freedom to state anger.

Some feelings are **combination** feelings. Emotions such as confused or frustrated are examples of two feelings coming together. Ask the client to identify which of the core feelings have combined to make "frustrating" or "confused." For example, frustration could be combinations of the feelings angry and helpless. Check it out.

Many times the tendency is to explain our feeling rather than to name it. Phrases like: *"I feel **that**, or I feel **like** . . ."* are **thoughts** about the feeling. The point, again, is not to figure out **why** I feel something, but to **simply name the feeling.**

When a client's check-in is **inconsistent** with his affect, **pointing out the discrepancy** can be useful.

Example: *"You are describing feeling happy, and I notice you are wringing your hands and that your outside looks like some anger might be going on. Can you go under the happy feelings to see if other feelings may be there too?"* The work of helping clients identify feelings can be tedious and feel nitpicky. However, it is invaluable to the alcoholic to know **exactly** what they're feeling and be able to clearly *"check in"* emotionally with others.

3. **Spiritual Check in:** *"The spiritual check in describes your relation to "God as you understand Him," or your Higher Power. If you are uncertain about God or a Higher Power, describe how you feel in your relation to the world. Do you have a sense of purpose, of belonging, of becoming awake?"*

4. **Setting a Goal: The second part of the check in is to** set a realistic, reachable goal for the day. **This goal** should be measurable **so that at the end of the day you can review it and know whether you completed the goal or not.**

At the end of the day, if you find you did not meet the goal, it is important information. You can reflect on what happened, or decide that the goal was unrealistic and could not be accomplished in a day. **The goal needs to be specific and include the action to meet it.** For instance: *"I will do four pages on my Step One, I will call my lawyer, and I will speak at the AA meeting tonight".*

Here is an example of a vague goal: *"I will just get through the day."*

"We have all managed to get through every day so far! What action will you take to get through the day sober? If your goal is not clear, the group again will help you to be more specific."

Note:
If a client is stuck on a goal, you may suggest this: *"Do you need to talk about how you are feeling emotionally? Could this be your goal for the day? How will you do that?"* If he cannot come up with a plan, suggest: *"Would talking about it in group therapy be useful?"*

The client must identify his own feelings and goals. Group members suggesting how someone else feels or what they should do repeats past intrusive behavior to the client. This also permits the client to be passive.

Staff can role model the check-in, without being over disclosing:

Example:

"Physically, I feel tired. My energy is low and I'm yawning a lot. Emotionally, I feel anxious and excited. Spiritually, I feel grateful and safe. My goal for today is to work with the group on the disease concept of alcoholism, and to call my shrink to see if 20 years of working with alcoholics has made me a nut!"

HANDOUT # 16

FEELING VOCABULARY

Warm	Gutsy	Spunky	Defeated	Delighted
Watched	Suspect	Important	Masculine	Disappointed
Judged	Needed	Unneeded	Rejected	No Good
Cared For	Protected	Secure	Hopeless	Light
Lost	Inadequate	Feminine	Disgusted	Used
Rewarded	Appreciated	Unrewarded	Empty	Jumpy
Stopped	Cornered	Risky	Virile	Put Down
Inferior	Childish	Indifferent	Seen	Guilty
Ignored	Unseen	Cuddled	Despised	Startled
Frisky	Helpless	Useless	Giddy	Endless
Childlike	Sunny	Timid	Loved	Bold
Unnoticed	Overloaded	Humiliated	Withdrawn	Serene
Grieved	Poor Me	Avoided	Relieved	Cloudy
Hazy	Strong	Happy	Enduring	Sad
Lonely	Desperate	Powerful	Tough	Confident
Pitiful	Bright	Let Down	Babied	Spiritual
Repaid	Despondent	Close	Stepped On	Weak
Alone	Calm	Quiet	Left Out	Grateful
Foolish	Ashamed	Hopeful	Jittery	Empty
Forced	Trapped	Dejected	Funny	Whole
Shy	Gloomy	Pleasant	Cocky	Content
Tender	Joyous	Peaceful	Captivated	Unhappy
Wounded	Hurt	Martyred	Impish	Attracted
Positive	Complete	Fulfilled	Clumsy	Buoyant
Longing	Heavy	Sprightly	Stingy	Lively
Crushed	Alarmed	Horrified	Dour	Refreshed
Brave	Washed Out	Carefree	Icy	Craving
Needy	Frustrated	Terrified	Unwanted	Scared
Beaten	Frantic	Turned Away	Satisfied	Frightened
Walked On	Tranquil	Irritated	Annoyed	Ridiculed
Humble	Powerless	Jealous	Challenged	Compassionate
Cold	Holy	Despondent	Embarrassed	

ASSERTIVENESS TRAINING

Passive, aggressive, and passive/aggressive behaviors keep us from true honesty, openness, and willingness. Learning and practicing assertive behavior is the most direct route to recovery.

Individual Goal: Clients will understand the concepts of passive, aggressive, passive/aggressive, and assertive behaviors in relation to their recovery.

Group Goal: Clients are given the opportunity to disclose their own behaviors and identify the behaviors of their peers.

Presentation: There are many ways to categorize behavior. For example: Positive and negative behaviors, constructive and destructive behaviors, healthy and unhealthy behaviors, etc. *In this presentation we will look at behaviors in terms of action.* We do this because a recovery program is a ***"program of action."***

The goal of this presentation is to understand and practice assertive behavior.

Assertiveness refers to the action of **expression of personal needs and rights without compromising or subtracting from the legitimate needs of others.** It means "standing in my boots." It is about owning and expressing thoughts and feelings directly and spontaneously, standing up for one's rights and asking for one's needs or wants. To assert oneself is to "put yourself forward," sometimes into the unknown. It is an equality of power, not domination, not submission and not manipulation.

In order to stay sober it is imperative that we learn to stand up for ourselves in difficult and high pressure situations.

Most of us have developed less effective ways of expressing ourselves and getting our needs met. Changing this behavior can be awkward and somewhat scary. But **If I always do what I've always done, I'll always get what I've always got.**

PASSIVE BEHAVIOR

Passive or non-assertive behavior is basically the choice on **non-action.** This behavior is **avoidant** and **indirect**. Protection of rights and attainment of needs are left to others.

Brainstorm with the group — What does passive behavior look like?

Example:

Quiet	Sweet	No direct eye contact
Weak	Mild	Speech is hesitant or minimal
Shy	Inhibited	Sitting with head down
Introverted		

Often it is helpful if the counselor physically models passive behavior. Passive behavior is just one step away from "one-arm curls."

Mime solitary isolated drinking, sitting with head down,and shoulders forward.

Explain to the group that most of us know passive behavior only too well. Because recovery is an inside job, ask the group members to stand and assume a passive body stance. See if they can determine what passive behavior **feels** like emotionally.

Tell them to take their time.

Give the group a minute or two to experience a passive stance. Now, ask them to shake it off.

What feelings came up for them?

Often heard responses include: Lonely, sad, weak, less than, isolated, wanting the world to disappear, poor me.

Poor me, poor me, pour me a drink.

Overall, passive behavior seems uncomfortable. *But there are payoffs to this behavior or we wouldn't do it.*

What are some of the advantages to passive behavior?

Doing nothing can keep us from making a mistake.
Not to risk is to play it safe.
Others won't be afraid.
It's easy.
You won't get into trouble.
Lets other people do the work.
There are times when to say nothing is the best choice.

We have gotten a lot of positive reinforcement to be passive as children.

For example: *"She's so good and sweet, she never gives me any trouble." "He's a good boy, he never cries." "Children should be seen and not heard." "We all like him, he's so easy going."*

Our goal is not to eliminate passive behavior. Rather it is to make it a choice.

In summary, although passive behavior can work for you it can also work against you.

Passive Behaviors:

Avoids problems.
Establishes a pattern of others taking advantage of you.
Lets others guess how you think and feel.
Lets others choose for you.
Destroys self-confidence.
Keeps you small and unimportant.
Builds anger and resentment.
Plays the victim.

AGGRESSIVE BEHAVIOR

On the other end of the spectrum is **aggressive** behavior. Aggresive is dominating. It insists on needs being met and imposes rights at the expense of others. **Aggression is an invasion on the rights, needs and feelings of others.** It can be *physical* or *verbal.*

Brainstorm with the group to determine what aggressive behavior looks like.

Example:

Angry	Strong	Staring or glaring eye contact
Rude	Loud	Bossy
Swearing	Direct	Puts others down
Threatening	Demanding	Dangerous

Model this behavior for the group.

Very energetically, jaws tight, scowling, glaring, finger pointing and fist clenching loudly demand that a client give you their pencil or notebook. It is important to keep a sense of playfulness so as to not become too threatening or truly frightening. At the same time, really try to get the pencil!

Thank the client for playing along with you and return the pencil. Ask the group to describe what they saw.

Example:

An angry person.
Someone who got what he/she wanted, but at the expense of someone else.
Cocky, hostile behavior.
Someone who views his/her rights as superior to others.
Overtly controlling behavior.
Victimizes others.

Aggressiveness is pushing and barreling through for what you want regardless of the rights or feelings of others. Aggression can be either physical or verbal.

Many of us operate out of these behaviors. Not drinking we can be peaceful, gentle people, maybe even overly so. After drinking we can have a complete behavioral change becoming violent, cruel, or emotionally abusive. It does not hold true for everyone, however.

"How many of you can identify a personality change from relatively passive to aggressive behavior while drinking or hungover?"

Ask for specific examples of verbal and nonverbal agressive behaviors. We have the ability to change our behaviors in sobriety. We choose our behaviors. They don't run us.

PASSIVE /AGGRESSIVE BEHAVIOR

A more complex behavior is the combination of passive and aggressive behaviors. It is called, not surprisingly, **passive/aggressive behavior.** Another name for this behavior is *"manipulating"* behavior. Passive/Aggressive behavior is manipulating, deceitful, and indirect. This behavior appears *passive on the outside,* but is *aggressive on the inside.*
This behavior attacks the integrity of others.

What does this type of behavior look like?

Deceptive
Sarcastic
Sneaky
Fake, phony
Uses "put downs"
Sly fox
Goes "around the bush"
Condescending
Talks about others, rather than being direct
Gossips

Passive/aggressive behavior is the behavior of a *hidden agenda*. It is *conning* behavior. A con man sees his "mark" as inherently stupid, less than, but behaves in a friendly humble way. **The outside behavior does not match the inside.**

Example:

Outside	**Inside**
"Honest, I'll try really hard."	"I'm not going to do it."
"Thank you very much."	"***@#*!#*! you** very much".
"I'm okay."	"You're too stupid to ever understand how I feel".
"I don't know."	"Maybe I know, maybe I don't, but it's none of your business".

Passive/aggressive behavior can be subtle.

Examples:

Being habitually late.
Controlling others by making them wait.
Smiling all the time.
Being overly "nice."
Sarcastic put-downs. ("You're not **that** fat." "You are not **really** stupid.")

Passive/aggressive behavior carries a lot of pain. To be filled with anger and superiority can be a very lonely place. Thank goodness that while we may be powerless over our feelings, we are not powerless over our behavior. We can catch ourselves behaving passive/aggressively. ***We have a choice.***

ASSERTIVE BEHAVIOR

One choice we have is to behave **assertively. What does assertive behavior look like?**

Looks relaxed, confident
Loud enough
Direct eye contact
Open
Emotionally honest
Expressive
Strong

In assertive behavior:

The other person knows how you think and feel.
The problem is attacked, not the other person.
Talks to others with respect for that person and self.
Makes choices for self.
Establishes a pattern of respect for future dealings.

Sounds rational, doesn't it? And, yet, many of us have some beliefs that keep us from acting assertively. Here they are. Do you find them irrational?

Go over Handout # 17, "Commom Irrational Beliefs."

Hold a brief discussion.

HANDOUT #17

COMMON IRRATIONAL BELIEFS :

1. If I assert myself, others will become angry.

2. If I assert myself and people do become angry with me, I will be devastated, and it will be awful.

3. Although I prefer others to be straight forward with me, I'm afraid that if I'm open with others and say no, I will hurt them.

4. If my assertion hurts others, I am responsible for their feelings.

5. If I assert myself, others will not accept my behavior and reject me.

6. It is wrong and selfish to turn down legitimate requests. Other people will think I'm terrible and won't like me.

7. At all costs, I must avoid making statements and asking questions that make me look ignorant or stupid.

8. My feelings and point of view are not as important as those of others.

9. I need to respond quickly and forcefully in all situations.

10. If I am assertive, I will get into situations which are beyond my control.

11. I must be aggressive to prove that I am a man/woman.

12. If I express positive feelings to another and I am rejected, then I will be devastated and it will be awful.

ASSERTIVENESS — INTO ACTION

This is the second half of the Assertiveness presentation. It is an opportunity for the group to synthesize what they learned during the lecture with what they already knew about their own behavior. It is a chance to practice assertiveness in recovery situations.

PART I:

Review these concepts with the group:

Point out to the group that **feelings** are separate from **behaviors**. Feelings can seduce our choices in behavior.

Example:

> With **passive behavior** comes **feelings** of safety, non-involvement, peace, rest, etc.
>
> With **aggressive behavior** comes **feelings** of power, strength, self righteousness, etc.
>
> With **passive/aggressive behavior** comes **feelings** of superiority, safety, self-righteous, etc.
>
> With **assertive behavior** comes **feelings** of dignity, self-worth, humanness, etc.

It can really feel terrific to punch someone in the nose. It can feel very awkward to let someone else know who we really are and how we feel.

In recovery, it is important to listen to and acknowledge our feelings and at the same time make conscious choices about our behaviors. The AA slogan, "Think, Think, Think" helps us remember this. Many times people will respond to why they relapsed with *"I don't know, I just felt like it."*

Thought before action.

A key to identifying our feelings **before** we make a behavioral decision is the following sentence:

When you________ , I feel ________.

Practice identifying feelings with the group by filling in the blanks with hypothetical feelings and actions. We are responsible for our feelings by our actions. **No one can make us feel any one way.** It means that: *No one can make us evil. No one can make us violent.*

Example:

A child who wants to go to the fair may feel sad when it rains. A farmer, during a drought period, may feel relieved or happy when it rains. **It is the same rain.**

This concept holds significant value for us as recovering people. It means that:

No one can make us drink.
No one can make us violent.

If your group members can fully accept this idea, it can give them a tremendous freedom.

Many of us behave out of habit. "If it worked once, it will work again." Some define insanity as ***doing the same thing over and over while expecting different results.*** We don't do this because we are stupid or insensitive people. It is our blind spots that keep us in behavioral ruts.

PART II:

The following exercise will help clarify the four types of behavior and give us the opportunity to use the AA tool of "acting as if . . ."

Example:

For a naturally shy and quiet person, to act assertively may feel "over-the-top" or aggressive.
For a naturally aggressive person to act assertively may feel weak or passive.

The object of this role play exercise is to Guess The Behavior.

Materials needed: Props for role plays: Laundry detergent box, plastic cups, extra chairs, a copy of the AA preamble, *How It Works,* and the 12 Traditions of AA read in meetings. A blackboard to highlight conceptual points.

1. Ask for a review of each behavior described in the lecture.

   A. **Assertive Behavior** — Standing up for ourselves without putting other people down.

B. **Passive Behavior** — Laid back, quiet. Does not take a stand.

C. **Aggressive Behavior** — Pushing our wants or needs on others, regardless of their feelings.

D. **Passive/Aggressive Behavior** — Manipulates others to get what we want.

2. Ask for examples of specific behaviors from the group's experience in each behavior. What did it feel like?

   Often clients will respond with what they expect you to hear.

   Examples: "I was assertive last night at the meeting when I raised my hand and I felt really good about myself."

   "I was aggressive when I punched out my friend. I felt guilty."

Contract with the group for non-violence during the activity. It can be tempting to really act out when one is encouraged to act aggressively.

Role play situation #1: A person returns a box of laundry detergent to the customer service representative of a large store without a receipt. The policy of the store is to give no refunds or exchanges without a receipt. This policy is inflexible. No behavior will warrant a refund or exchange. As recovering people we are responsible for the action, not the outcome.

The clients play the dissatisfied customers and the counselor plays (for at least two role plays) the customer service representative.

Acknowledge the client who agrees to take on the first role play. That action is assertive in itself. Applause can serve as reinforcement for people who take personal risks.

Secretly decide with the client what behavior (passive, aggressive, etc) each of you will demonstrate.

Begin the scene.

After the scene has been played out, ask the group which behavior they saw played out. Some may be obvious and other role plays more obscure. It is important to be sensitive to the clients playing the dissatisfied customers. To get up before the group is to take a risk. Repeat the same situation with different clients acting out different behaviors.

Review this idea with the group:

- *People behave in different ways in different situations.*

Example:

A prize fighter may be the ideal example of aggressive behavior in the boxing ring and remain totally passive in front of his domineering parents.

How is your behavior different in different situations?

It is important that we practice assertive behavior in our recovery. What do we do in difficult situations affecting our recovery? It is one thing to plan your behavior with a counselor and quite another to consciously practice assertive behavior in a surprise situation.

The following are **surprise role plays.**
Ask for volunteers before the situation is disclosed.

Situation #2: Four clients are needed. Three using people pressure you to join them in relapse. You are alone in your own home and they knock on the door. Direct the three users to "play it to the hilt! How do you assert yourself?

Situation #3: Three clients are needed. You are one day out of treatment. Your old friends come over for a visit. Although they are well-meaning, they treat you as a complete invalid or are nervous around you. How do assert yourself?

Situation #4: Four clients are needed. Your new sponsor has agreed to go to coffee with you after a meeting. After the meeting you notice her laughing and joking and appearing to leave with two friends. How do you assert yourself?

Situation #5: Entire group. Ask the group to recreate an AA meeting. Ask clients to play the secretary and the group speaker. The secretary chooses peers to read the section, "How It Works" from Chapter 5 and the 12 Traditions.

Secretly choose a client to play an obnoxious, aggressive, intoxicated alcoholic. This role can also be played by another staff member. *The acting objective is to completely shut down the meeting.*

The scene: The meeting begins and the speaker begins his/her qualification. The obnoxious player enters and disrupts the meeting.

Questions for discussion might include: How much obnoxious behavior are you willing to put up with? How can the active alcoholic best be helped? What behavior did you exhibit during the interruption?

After the discussion, replay the scene.

In closing the presentations it is important to bring the group together. An applause acknowledgment or group confidentiality statement can bring the group back to a unit.

Ask the group to form a circle and make a group confidentiality statement.

We have taken some big risks today. My risks are mine. I agree that I am free to share my experience, but not that of the other people here. I state my name as agreement that what went on in the group will stay in the group.

Each member states their name. Break.

HANDOUT #18

ASSERTIVENESS

As a person I have a right to:

1. Be treated with respect.
2. Have and express my own feelings and opinions. **"When you____ , I feel ____.**
3. Be listened to and taken seriously.
4. Set my own priorities.
5. Say no without feeling guilty.
6. Ask for what I want.
7. Make mistakes — and be responsible for them.
8. Be uncertain or uncommitted as to what I want, and need time to make decisions.
9. Ask for information and/or support from professionals, family, and friends when I feel I want it (even though I may be turned down).
10. Say "I don't have the answer."
11. Say "I need some time to think that over."
12. Have my needs be as important as the needs of others.
13. Change my mind.
14. Grow, learn, and change.
15. Feel and express anger.
16. Be competent and be proud of my accomplishments.

17. Say "I don't understand."

18. Say "I don't agree."

19. Be myself.

20. Choose not to assert myself.

Assertive behavior means standing up for what I think and feel while respecting the rights of others.

UNDERSTANDING BOUNDARIES

We all have personal boundaries.

Our boundary defines who we are and determines how we are able to interact and relate to the world, physically, emotionally, and spiritually.

My boundary lets me know where I end and you begin.

My boundary allows me to express who I am and allows you to do the same.

If we grew up in a dysfunctional family, inconsistency and various forms of abuse influenced our ability to form and maintain our boundaries. We also have difficulty identifying the boundaries of others.

Damaged boundaries is another symptom of codependency.

The primary cause of conflict and difficulties in relationships lies in unhealthy boundaries. My boundary is my container. When I am too contained or not contained enough, then problems in relationships result.

Healing and restoring our boundary is a part of the recovery process. It does not happen overnight.

Our **physical boundary** sets our need and right to physical space and safety; including our needs and rights in sexual interaction with others.

Our **emotional** or **internal boundary** sets our emotional needs, rights, and safety; including our right to our thoughts and actions.

If I develop an **overly protective boundary,** my ability to be in healthy relationships with others is compromised. It is like being surrounded physically and emotionally by a steel capsule. *Nothing can penetrate in or out.* The give and take, back and forth flow in a relationship is hampered.

The other extreme is **a lack of a sense of boundary.** I cannot experience myself as separate from others. My container is faulty and all the contents spill out just like an egg when the shell is broken. *It becomes difficult to distinguish myself from others.* I feel my feelings and all of your feelings too. I begin to define myself according to your definition. I lose my own identity. *My feelings are your feelings, my thoughts are your thoughts, and I behave the way I think you want me to.*

A **healthy boundary** is like the permeable membrane of a cell. *It controls what goes in and out*. It determines what it needs and goes for it. There is a back and forth flow.

As our self-esteem increases in recovery, so will the health of our boundaries.

Let's look in greater detail at some of the characteristics of damaged boundaries.

Materials needed: Blackboard

1. Before beginning this part of the group, place this information the blackboard:

    Physical Boundary: Governs our need and right to physical space and safety; including needs and rights in sexual interaction with others.

    Emotional Boundary: Governs our emotional needs and rights, and safety; including our right to our thoughts and behavior.

2. Draw these diagrams:

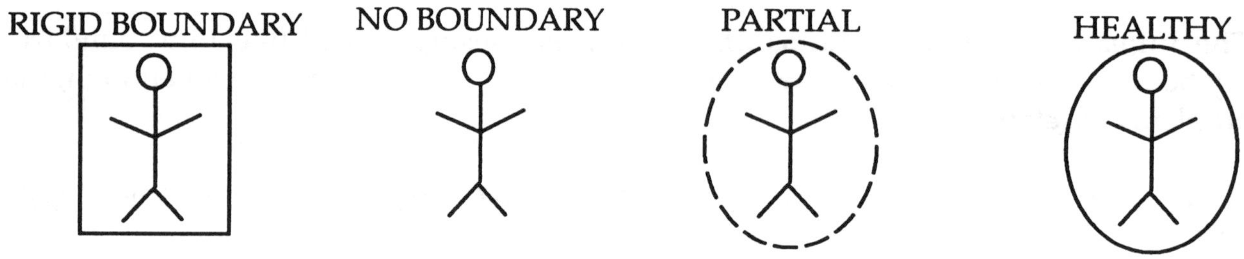

3. Review and discuss these diagrams with the group:

    - **The rigid boundary** is like an impenetrable wall. Nothing can go in or come out.
    - **No boundary -** The person is unprotected. Everything can flood in and flood out.
    - **Partial boundaries** work sometimes but are not reliable.
    - **Healthy boundaries** protect the individual, and the person can choose what comes in and goes out.

4. Distribute Handouts #19 and #20, "Descriptions Of Boundaries". Review the items in each section, asking for identification and examples from group members.

5. Lastly, distribute the Handout #21, "My Boundaries". Discuss the responses in a follow-up group, or at the beginning of the next group, *"Physical And Emotional Boundaries"*.

HANDOUT #19

DESCRIPTIONS OF BOUNDARIES

RIGID BOUNDARIES:

Physical:

Stiff body posture.
Stoic.
Uncomfortable being touched.
Avoids touching or showing affection to others.
Avoids physical closeness.
Does not react or under-reacts.
"Stone face".
Very predictable behavior.

Emotional:

Appears insensitive to the feelings of others.
Appears aloof and disinterested.
Does not show feelings.
Does not talk about feelings.
Seems emotionally numb.
Attempts to meet needs and wants by themselves.
Has difficulty asking for or accepting help from others.
Does not react or under-reacts emotionally.
Has difficulty giving or receiving from others.

NO BOUNDARIES:

Physical:

Does not like being alone.
Touches others without asking.
Allows others to touch him/her even when it is uncomfortable or inappropriate.
Is not aware of own need for privacy.
Imposes on the privacy of others.
Allows physical space to be invaded.
Over-reacts to the feelings and behavior of others.
Personalizes.
Behavior is influenced by others.
Is unpredictable.

Emotional:

Feels everything.
Feels the feelings of others.
Cannot contain feelings.
Over-discloses, tells too much.
Is dependent on others for emotional well-being.
Gets too close too fast.
Feels like a victim.
Experiences prolonged resentments.
Is overwhelmed and preoccupied with others.
Says yes when he/she wants to say no.
Feels responsible for the feelings of others.
Identity tied to being in an intimate relationship.
Overcompensates.
Expects others to meet needs.
Gives too much.
Takes too much.
Unable to respect the rights of others.

PARTIAL BOUNDARIES:

Physical:

May have extremes in need for physical space.
Shows characteristics of fluctuation in boundaries.
May have rigid or healthy boundaries in some circumstances and fragile boundaries in others.

Emotional:

Has mood swings.
Is indirect —
Example: Shares feelings about marriage with mother rather than with husband.
Is emotionally inconsistent. — May have rigid or healthy boundaries in some circumstances and fragile boundaries particularly in intimate relationships.

HEALTHY BOUNDARIES

Physical:

Makes physical boundary clear to others.
Respects and is sensitive to the needs and rights of others.
Is able to negotiate and compromise.
Asks permission before touching others.

Emotional:

Shares feelings appropriately and directly.
Is assertive .
Is interdependent.
Identifies choices.
Is able to make mistakes without damage to self-esteem.
Has an internal sense of personal identity.
Can allow "differentness" in others.
Tolerates and accepts differences of opinion without altering their own.
Is sensitive to feelings of others (empathetic).

HANDOUT #20

Other Signs Of Unhealthy Boundaries:

Sexual:

Having sex when you do not want to.
Falling in love at first sight.
Intimate sharing on first meeting.
Using sex as a reward or punishment.
Inability to distinguish between love and sex.
Manipulating another person through sex.
Feeling a need to always be in a sexual relationship.
Attaching self-esteem to sexual attraction.
Forcing sex on someone who does not want it.
Sexual abuse.

Physical:

Touching others without asking.
Physical intimidation.
Not allowing others privacy.
Not protecting your own need for privacy.
Physical abuse.

Emotional:

Verbal abuse.
Making threats.
Assuming I know what someone else feels.
Assuming others know what I feel.
Expecting others to know my needs and meet them.
Assuming to know the needs of others.
Over-reaction to feelings or behavior of others.
Insisting others tell us how they feel.
Not respecting the rights of others.
Intolerance to differences in opinion.
Dependence on others for my sense of well-being.
Inability to ask for help.
Personalizing.
Need for constant reassurance from others.
Going against personal values and morals to please others.

Unclear about preferences.
Accepting gifts that I don't want.
Making material gifts the measure of another's caring.
Over giving.
Frequent advice-giving with expectation that others follow it.

HANDOUT #21

MY BOUNDARIES

What kind of boundary do I have?

Where in my life is it the hardest to have a healthy boundary?

What changes would I like to make in my boundary?

What do I need to do to make these changes?

PHYSICAL AND EMOTIONAL BOUNDARIES

Introduction: After the group "Understanding Boundaries", clients have the theoretical framework of boundaries. They "get it" intellectually. This group helps them "get it" emotionally, which makes the theoretical framework real. These groups use action method to create a personal experience, to concretize the concept of boundaries.

PHYSICAL BOUNDARIES EXERCISE :

Physical or external boundaries: This is a simple and effective exercise to demonstrate physical boundaries. Ask for a volunteer from the group, Joe.

1. Stand and face the client with at least 15 to 20 feet between you.

2. *Directions to the group:* "Joe and I are going to find our physical boundary with each other. First, I will walk slowly up to Joe, making eye contact. I will walk up to a point where I feel **uncomfortably** close, and then back up to the place I feel **comfortable. This distance is my physical boundary with Joe."**

3. *Demonstrate for the group.* Have Joe now repeat the exercise.

4. Ask the group to break up into pairs and to do the exercise.

Discussion:

Could you feel your comfort zone, your physical boundary?

Does every one have the same boundary?

If one person needs more space than the other, whose boundary takes precedence?

Our boundary does not remain the same with everyone. Our emotional condition can also impact on the space we need. If I'm angry with you do I need more or less space? If you are angry with me, do I need more or less space?

The physical boundary involves at least two people. **How can we assert our need for space?**

Examples:

- Back up if someone is too close.
- Tell someone, "You are a little too close. This is uncomfortable for me."

Our boundary is unconsciously invaded all the time and we unknowingly invade the boundaries of others. Our reactions can vary.

Demonstration: Set up two chairs, one behind the other. Ask for a volunteer. Have this person sit in the chair in front. Set up a scenario:

You are in an AA meeting. You sit in one chair and put your foot on the chair of the client. Be annoying, tap your foot on the chair, accidentally tap your foot against the client, saying "Excuse me".

Ask the client, "What do you do?"

Have the group join in with how they would react. Have them note their emotional reaction.

Clarify the problem. *This person has their foot on my chair and I am uncomfortable with it.* Have I reacted by invading the other person's boundary in retaliation? Have I sat there getting madder and madder and building up resentment? Is there a simple way of resolving this problem?

Switch chairs with the client. Have him demonstrate the intrusive behavior. Respond to him assertively.

Example:

> "Excuse me, when you put your foot on my chair, I feel uncomfortable. Will you please take it down? Thank you." Is the original problem solved?

Let's look at how we have invaded the physical boundaries of others and how others invade ours.

Make two columns on the board: Generate a list from the group:

Ways My Boundary is Invaded	**Ways I Invade Others**
People Hugging me in AA.	Sitting on John's lap without asking.
Peers in treatment touching me without asking.	Pinching a peer during a lecture.

It is **my responsibility** to let others know what my boundary is. Usually people are responsive to me.

Note: Physical abuse is always an invasion of boundaries. A history of using violence against others needs to be addressed in discharge planning. Framing the abusive behavior as a boundary violation is a non-shaming way to begin the work.

EMOTIONAL: INTERNAL BOUNDARIES

INTRODUCTORY NOTES TO CLINICIAN:

Emotional boundaries are the most important part of the boundaries work. It's where our clients are the most wounded and have the most difficulty meeting their needs. It is also the most difficult aspect of the boundaries group to explain.

We have found that even the best clinical definitions of emotional or internal boundaries still leaves our clients confused about what they mean. The most effective teaching method is to **demonstrate** emotional boundaries, explaining "what just happened" during and after the demonstration.

Example:

"My emotional boundary is like a balloon **around** my feelings inside."

For example: "I wake up . It's a beautiful day. I made love to my boyfriend. He said he loved me for the first time in months."

"Inside me", **point to your solar plexus,** "I feel these wonderful feelings. It's like light helium inside a balloon"

With both hands create a balloon in front of you for the group to see and say:

"The balloon is my **boundary**. It **contains** my feelings. The balloon is my internal boundary. **It is separate from my feelings.** The boundary allows the feelings to get larger or smaller. My feelings fill the space in my solar plexus."

Point and lightly rub your solar plexus again.

"My boyfriend goes off to work. I'm so in love with him. I do the laundry. I empty out his pant's pocket. A note falls out, I don't recognize the writing. It says "Darling, I so enjoyed sleeping with you again yesterday. When will you tell your girlfriend that you're moving out? You promised to do it today!"

Clutch your solar plexus, demonstrate a look of shock or pain, slump your shoulders down.

Look at the group and inform them:

*" **My balloon burst. I have just lost my internal boundary.** That happy feeling has just evaporated."*

Process with the group.
What just happened? This is obviously an extreme example but it makes its point. "My feelings are inside the boundary of the balloon. I feel light and happy."

Demonstrate the balloon again.

"Something from the outside comes in. I can't fight it off. *I have no protection.* It dive bombs my balloon and bursts the outside, **the boundary** of my inside feelings. My feelings spill all over my entire world. **Everything** has changed for me emotionally. *I can't control it.* "

Demonstrate an attack on the balloon.

"This is what we're talking about, but it happens on the inside of my body; my inside boundary.

For example, a more realistic example: "I show up at work, I'm in a great mood. It's a beautiful day. I'm wearing a cute dress and looking good." **Place your hand high on your chest and look happy.** "Mary here , rushes up to me and says "Have you seen the boss? He's looking for you." **Drop your hand down to your lower gut and look worried.** "I just lost my internal boundary. I'm getting fired. It's a horrible day. I look like a tramp."

"The problem with emotional boundaries, for most of us, is that we seem to have no control over them."

"There's nothing wrong with my feelings." **Point to your abdomen.**

"The problem was my **head.**" **Point to your head.** "I heard Mary and *automatically assumed* that I would be fired. What if my boss was really going to offer me a raise? A promotion?"

"There is something funny up here in my head, **my filtering system** which destroyed my internal boundary and my feelings churned up."

"The other problem was that I have *only one boundary* around **all** of my feelings. My boundary included my job security, how I felt about my day and how I felt I looked. Because I have all **of the parts of myself clumped together**, when my boundary is threatened, *everything goes* . "

"Some people can worry about their jobs, yet their day is still beautiful and they know they still look darned cute in their dress. ***They've been able to form separate boundaries to influence separate issues* . "**

This is what we'll be looking at today:

What kind of filters do I have?
What kind of emotional boundaries do I have?
How do I set healthy boundaries so my balloon isn't always exploding or my insides dropping down by outside events?
How do I keep the rest of my boundaries if one of them collapses - keep the rest of my day and my self-esteem intact?
How do I maintain feeling OK if the outside world seems crazy?
How do I check out the reality of the outside world so I'm not falsely affected by it?

EMOTIONAL : INTERNAL BOUNDARIES

In exploring emotional boundaries, we need to remember a few points. Our internal, emotional boundary has a filter. The filter is in our head. Our head determines what information will be allowed in and what will be revealed from the inside. This filter monitors what we think and what we do.

In relationships, other people reflect to us what they know about us. A healthy filter tells us whether they are correct or not, and allows us to put out the information they need to see us clearly.

For most of us, our filter has been battered and torn, and has lost its effectiveness. In recovery, we can begin to repair the damage.

Let's begin by taking a look at how and what information we take in from others.

Any information must be evaluated first by the filter in our heads. We don't want to take in anything that is incorrect and does not fit or belong to us, but we need to acknowledge it if it does.

So first, we must determine if the information we receive is true or not. If it is accurate, we allow the information in through the appropriate emotional boundary to our feelings and respond. If it is not true, we do not let it through the filter to our emotions, and we let the other person know this is not true for us. Sometimes making a clear determination requires that we have more information.

Example:

My partner asks to talk to me. She says, *"I'm worried. You haven't talked to me in three days. This is how you acted when you were drinking. Are you drinking?"*

Healthy Boundary: I think: ***"It is true that I have been isolating for three days.*** *I have not been drinking."* **I feel** accepting of what is said. **I respond:** *"You're right about the isolation. I've been feeling bored and lonely. I haven't been drinking. I am sorry if I have ignored you. Let's go out for dinner tonight."*

Rigid or Over-protective Boundary: I think: ***"None of this is true,*** *"She worries about everything."* **I feel** defensive. **I respond:** *"You're worried about nothing."*

Absent or Under-protective Boundary: I think: ***"Everybody hates me."*** **I feel** hurt or angry. **I respond:** *"How can you ask that? You don't trust me. I'm trying so hard and all you do is criticize me. No wonder I don't want to talk to you!"*

In the last two examples, the information was not evaluated completely or accurately. I discounted or judged my partner's reality and did not take responsibility for my own.

The way in which we receive and give information can also influence our filter.

When we perceive attacks on our thinking, feelings, beliefs, or behavior, we tend to block out information, and take a defensive stance.

In healthy boundaries we focus on ourselves. We own what we think, feel, and believe. We own what we do. We also define actions we will take to assertively maintain our boundaries or space.

The following format is a simple way to express when we are affected by someone else's behavior. (We want to be heard. We want to avoid placing the other person in a place of defense.)

"When you ________________, I feel ______________. I need _____________.

If you (continue to) ________________, I will ____________ ."

Example:

"My friend invited me to a movie. She called at the last minute to cancel. I was really looking forward to going out. This is the third time in the last two weeks that she has canceled plans."

Healthy Boundary: "**When you** repeatedly make plans with me and cancel, **I feel** angry, hurt, and annoyed. **I need** you to follow through when we have plans to go out. **If you** cancel again, **I will** not make any more plans with you."

Unhealthy Boundary: Response: "You are totally unreliable. I do not know why I bother with you at all." This type of response **puts others on the defensive**. (Blaming.)

Unhealthy Boundary: "It's okay if you have something more important to do. After all, what are friends for?" This response is **passive. I do not get my needs met.**

In the first example, healthy boundaries , notice that I make an observation, own my feelings, and clearly present my needs to the other person. Consider that almost all the conflict we have in relationships are over boundaries.

What are repeated conflicts that come up in your relationships?

Let's use this format to address some of them and see if it makes a difference.

Using the format above, explore some examples from the group.

Help them separate their issues and emotional boundaries so they can see how to have a "good" day if one boundary collapses.

SEXUALITY

Talking about sex can be uncomfortable for most of us. In our society and in many of our families, it is a taboo subject. Many of us deal with sexuality through humor. Just think of all the "dirty jokes" we've told and heard over the years. For many of us this is a mask for the discomfort and confusion we have experienced about our sexuality. We are the most vulnerable in sexual relationships, no matter how we might try to disguise it. Most of us are not educated about sex and so take many misconceptions about sex to the bed room with us.

Our sexual identities have been shaped and fashioned by the stereotyped roles and attitudes presented to us by society, religion, and family. They color what we should do, how we should do it, and how we should look as sexual beings. Sexuality can't follow rules and roles, *it just is,* so many of us experience a sense of failure by not measuring up to these notions. This can leave us confused, guilty, and ashamed.

Reasons For Sex:

Procreation
Bonding
Pleasure

The Impact Of Chemical Dependency On Sexuality:

Initially our use of chemicals can decrease sexual anxiety and inhibitions. However, over time these same chemicals can affect our performance and judgment in sexual relationships.

Prolonged chemical use for men can cause neurological difficulties in erection, premature ejaculation and impotence. For men and women, prolonged use of chemicals also affects hormonal balances. In women, this may be experienced as changes in the menstrual cycle (See Medical Aspects). For both sexes, chronic use effects libido.

Men and women both have shame related to poor judgment around their sexual behavior. This shame increases and has a negative impact on their feelings of self-esteem and self-worth. Sexual recovery must be addressed as an integral part of treatment.

Some of the issues we need to explores as part of sexual recovery are:

Sexual Identity
Sexual Boundaries
Homosexuality/Bisexuality
Concerns About Sexually Transmitted Disease
Sexual Abuse
Pregnancy
Abortion
Child Birth
Menopause
Impotence
Prostate Problems

We frequently hear in the program that "We are as sick as our secrets." For most of us, our greatest secrets revolve around sex. We keep secret those things which cause us the most shame. Working with a sponsor or therapist and working the 4th and 5th Steps, helps us resolve our shame and reveal our secrets. The only way to heal the shame within us is to allow others to know about our pain and receive the nurturing we lacked.

Ask the group to review messages they have received about sex, sexuality, and gender roles. Write them on the blackboard.

MESSAGES:

Sex is dirty.

Don't talk about sex, just do it.

Men should take the lead in sex.

The sole purpose of sex is procreation.

Women don't make sexual advances.

It is the woman's duty to always be available sexually to her man.

Sex outside the marriage is a sin.

Man is the provider.

Men are the dominant sex.

Homosexuality is a perversion.

Women who don't experience orgasm are frigid.

Sexual Boundaries And Intimacy:

We live in a sexually dysfunctional society. The misconceptions, unrealistic expectations, and pressures associated with sexuality make defining our sexual identity confusing and difficult at best.

We have all been influenced by the Hollywood guidelines of what "sexy" looks and acts like. Let's face it folks, most of us are not "Tens". We are sexual beings, however, with sexual needs and desires and the capacity for attaining intimacy with others.

Sex and Intimacy are not the same thing. Sex is a physical interaction. Intimacy ("Into Me See") covers wider ground. Being intimate is about sharing who I am:

My thoughts, feelings, and beliefs.

My capacity to achieve intimacy with others is first dependent upon the development of my own identity and boundary. Increasing self awareness, self esteem and trust in who we are, will help us develop healthy sexual boundaries.

Being aware of unhealthy sexual boundaries can help us initiate changes in our sexual recovery. Sometimes it's easier to see what doesn't work rather than to see what does work. What are some signs of unhealthy sexual boundaries?

Make a list on the blackboard:

Involve the group by asking them to provide examples for each point.

UNHEALTHY SEXUAL BOUNDARIES:

Having sex when I don't want to.

Manipulating others through sex.

Inability to distinguish love from sex.

Sense of self-esteem tied to sexual relationship.

Discomfort discussing sex with partner.

Demanding sex from partner.

Sexual put down related to performance or physical appearance.

Sexual abuse.

Using sex as punishment or reward.

Falling in love at first sight.

Using sex as a means of avoiding conflict or to resolve conflict.

Indiscriminate sex as a way to relieve loneliness.

Irrational jealousy.

Inability To Express My Sexual Needs And Wants:

Most of us have the most difficulty maintaining our boundaries in sexual relationships.

Clarity on who we are sexually is an important part of recovery. We need to grow in touch with ourselves before we can be intimate with others.

Getting involved in new sexual relationships early in our recovery can take the focus off our personal growth and recovery program. I need to know who I am before I can share myself with someone else.

Review Handout #22 with the group. Spend time clarifying and discussing each point with the group.

A follow-up therapy group will allow clients to begin exploring individual sexual issues.

We only recommend **same sex groups** for this work.

You may use the list previously provided under "The Impact Of Chemical Dependency On Sexuality" for topics.

Identified issues of sexual abuse, sexual dysfunction, sexually transmitted disease, or pregnancy will need to be pursued by the clinician in discharge planning.

HANDOUT # 22

SEXUAL RECOVERY

Suggestions:

1. Get help for issues of sexual dysfunction. Most problems in sobriety are temporary. If they persist for greater than three to six months seek professional help.

2. Beware of using sex as a replacement addiction.

3. Practice assertiveness in your expression of sexual needs and preferences. Begin to own who you are sexually.

4. Be prepared for surfacing of tension and fears related to sex. They have been buried in alcohol and drugs for a long time for most of us. Talk about them if they arise.

5. Avoid the pressures of the performance and appearance traps. Doing the best we can with what we have got is good enough.

6. Own responsibility for your sexual behavior.

7. Be sensitive to the rights and needs of others.

8. Get the secrets out. Use your sponsor or a therapist. Place your secrets in a place that feels safe for you, so that you may begin to decrease feelings of shame.

9. If you are in a relationship with another recovering person, be sure to keep your programs separate.

10. Avoid the possibility of romance with a sponsor. Choose a sponsor who is not the gender of preferred sexual partners.

11. Work the 12 Steps of recovery.

AFFIRMATIONS

As addicts and alcoholics we have a disease. We are not bad and getting good. We are sick and getting better. In fact, we are already "good". Affirmations acknowledge our strengths and the beauty of sobriety.

Individual Goal: Hearing positive feedback is sometimes harder than hearing negative messages. Freedom from false pride and arrogance does not mean low self-esteem or self deprecating behaviors. Rather, true humility includes a willingness to fully accept our true selves, the facts of our lives and our openness to change.

Group Goal: Team building and relationships are developed as clients affirm each other's power and beauty.

Materials needed: Group room, black board, 3"x5" cards, writing materials.

Action: The counselor introduces the concept of affirming ourselves. To affirm is to say "Yes". An affirmation is a positive "Yes" statement. It is **not** conceit or show-off behavior. Rather, it is the beginning of positive self-esteem. Self-esteem must be learned and re-enforced to counter the negative messages of our lives.

1. Brainstorm with the group to identify the negative messages they have received from others. Comparing ourselves to others can also create feelings of low self-worth. We reinforce these messages ourselves.

Example:

"You're nothing but an alcoholic."
"You're stupid."
"You're worthless."
"You'll never amount to anything."
"Shut up."
"I'm hopeless."
"I'm ugly."
"I'm less than."

These negative messages, heard day after day contribute to low self-esteem.

2. Brainstorm with the group to establish what low self-esteem looks like.

Symptoms might include:

- Bragging or exaggerating — To give the impression we are okay.
- Perfectionism — "I am what I do."
- Not caring — Evidenced in dress, behavior, language, hygiene.
- Shyness or being a loner — "I don't have much to offer."
- Self-deprecating statements — Putting ourselves down.
- Being a follower or "people pleaser".
- Taking ridiculous risks —Setting ourselves up to fail or get hurt.
- Pretending to be someone else — "Wannabe's".
- Being overly critical —Putting others down to feel better about ourselves.
- Brushing off our accomplishments and compliments from others.

3. Ask for a volunteer, Mary, to stand before the group to receive positive feedback about her attributes.

   Ask the group to brainstorm to develop a list of this client's attributes. Emphasize that Brainstorming takes the form of complete sentences directed toward the client.

   For example: Instead of "*Brave*" or "*She is brave*", a complete message would be, "*Mary, you are brave.*"

4. Ask Mary to select another group member to record the affirming characteristics on a 3"x5" card.

5. Ask the group to make 8 - 10 affirming statements about Mary while you write them on the board beside her.

6. Ask Mary to circle three to four of the hardest qualities to accept.

7. The counselor takes the affirming qualities and writes a three to four sentence "I statement" affirmation on the blackboard.

   For example: Using the characteristics of "Brave, smart, caring, loving, good friend, kind strong, and funny" the counselor might write:

   "I, Mary, am a brave and loving woman. I have the inner strength to accept life on life's terms. I care deeply. I am sober today!"

   It is not necessary to use every positive attribute listed on the board. After all, it is only a partial list of all the wondrous qualities about Mary.

8. Give the client the opportunity to add to or edit the affirmation.

9. Instruct the client to read the affirmation to the group with feeling. Group applause.

10. The peer group member records the affirmation on the 3"x5" card.

    The affirmation card can be put in a convenient place to be seen and repeated on a daily basis (bathroom mirror, car dashboard, refrigerator, etc).

11. Ask the client to select a peer to receive the next affirmation. It is important that all group members are affirmed.

12. After all group members have received their positive statements, hold a discussion.

    What did it feel like to receive the caring from the group?
    What defenses do you use to keep from accepting your entire self?
    What will you do to make this affirmation a part of your recovery?

Suggestions and Pitfalls: It is important to keep the energy of the group high and the pace quick. This exercise has been designed for a small group of 8 to 10.

Variation: For a larger group, it is suggested that the group be broken down into pairs.

Each member of the pair lists the positive attributes of his/her partner.

The client uses these characteristics to create his/her own three to four sentence affirmation to be read before the group.

"I am a capable and qualified counselor. The work I am doing is important. I have the ability to roll with the punches. My heart and mind are open. I make a real difference!"

HANDOUT #23

AFFIRMATION

In the infinity of life where I am, all is perfect, whole and complete. The past has no power over me because I am willing to learn and to change. I see the past as necessary to bring me where I am today. I am willing to begin where I am right now to clean the rooms of my mental house. I know it does not matter where I start, so I now begin with the smallest and the easiest rooms, and in that way I will see the results quickly. I am thrilled to be in the middle of this adventure for I know I will never go through this particular experience again. I am willing to set myself free. All is well in my world.

LISTENING

Listening is one of the most powerful tools of sobriety. It takes practice. This presentation provides the opportunity to practice active listening and identification.

Individual Goal: To learn the value of listening, and truly hearing another recovering person's story and emotional life. Clients will recognize the importance of listening to the health inside us all.

Group Goal: Group cohesion is created through role reversals. The concept of listening is introduced to the group.

Presentation: *"Learn to listen and listen to learn."* Listening is a skill. Just as with any skill we all can get better at it. And, listening is a skill that can save our lives.

If we truly hear the experience of another person's recovery we can learn from it and apply it. Recovery is not about 'toughing it out on our own' in isolation. Rather, *it is about connecting with others.* ***Listening helps us do that.***

In this presentation we will be talking to and with each other.

Have you ever noticed two completely intoxicated people talking together? They seem to talk **at** each other, not **to** each other.

Brainstorm with the group. Have you ever had the experience of trying to communicate with someone and come away with the idea that they were not able to hear a word you said? What did it feel like? What did the other person's **not** listening look like?

We are able to listen with more than just our ears. We also listen with our eyes, our intuition, and our hearts. **What does listening look like?**

One of the most important parts of listening is identifying situations, and more importantly feelings, that we also have. ***Identifying means that for a brief moment we can imagine ourselves in the other person's situation.***

The Exercise: This exercise is one of listening and identifying. Ask the group members to divide themselves into pairs. If there is an odd number of people there will be one group of three. **Give out one "Listening Exercise" sheet to each pair.**

The sheet is intended as a catalyst for sharing. It is not necessary to write in the blanks because the responses may change from day to day, or moment to moment. It is also not necessary to get through every empty blank space.

Each pair finds a quiet place for each person, one at a time, to practice listening. Each person is given 5 minutes. The first person shares from the list. After five minutes, they switch and the second person shares while the other listens. At the end of 10 minutes, the pairs return to the group.

What was this experience like for you? Did you feel that your partner was able to hear you? Were you able to really listen to your partner? Did anything distract you? Is there anything you told your partner that you would not like the group to know? If so, let your partner know.

Ask for a volunteer pair to present their listening skills before the group. Instruct the two people to **reverse roles** with each other.

In order to reverse roles, the clients exchange chairs.
One client agrees to present first, Client A.
The other, Client B, stands behind Client A with their hands on Client A's shoulders.
Client A may use the "Listening Exercise" to prod her memory.
Client A presents the information that she heard from Client B.
After Client A has presented, ask Client B if he felt listened to.
Client B then takes Client A's empty seat and presents in the role reversal.

Repeat this format until all the pairs have presented.

In closing, affirm the group's willingness to take risks and to take on different roles. Briefly brainstorm with the group as to where they might best apply their listening skills.

HANDOUT #24

LISTENING EXERCISE

My name is________.

The reason I'm here is________.

Right now, I'm feeling_________.

When I'm in a new group, I_________.

When I'm in a new situation, I usually_________.

I'm happiest when________.

When I'm alone I usually_________.

My biggest worry, right now, is__________.

I get really angry when_________.

The way I'm feeling now is________.

I love________.

I feel a healthy pride when________.

I feel sad or blue when_________.

My feelings get easily hurt when_________.

I feel embarrassed when_________.

The last thing in the world I want to do is________.

The thing I like best about myself is________.

Toward you, right now, I feel________.

What I like best about you is_________.

What I like best about myself is__________.

Right now I'm feeling________.

MIRROR EXERCISE

Sobriety is an "inside job". The Mirror Exercise gives the clients the opportunity to look inside and share with a trusted peer. Intimacy can be seen as "Into Me See."

Individual Goal: To practice going within ourselves and to share this inside self with someone else. Who do I see when I look inside myself? Can I tell you who I really am?

Group Goal: A recognition that each person's recovery is special and particular. As group members *we can serve as mirrors for each other.*

Materials needed: A group room, a large mirror, an adjustable lamp. Handout #25 — "The Man In The Glass".

Action:

1. Group discussion to consider: What is it like to look at your reflection in the mirror? What do you see? What is the value of looking deeply into your own eyes?

2. Ask a group member to read "The Man In The Glass" to the group.

3. The action of this group will be to: "Just go to a mirror and look at yourself and see what that person has to say". Although it is a simple direction, to truly look deep within ourselves is not always easy.

4. The counselor writes two sentences on the board:

   "The way I see myself holding back is____."

   "The way I see myself growing is____."

   Ask the group to memorize these sentences, but not to fill in the blanks. The answer may come from the person in the glass.

5. Place the mirror in front of the room. The lamp is adjusted to illuminate the face of the client. Dim the lights of the room.

6. Instruct the clients to go to the mirror one at a time to *"see what that person has to say."*

Looking in the mirror, **really seeing** means getting past the externals (messy hair, a blemish, tired eyes, etc.). It is important to take the time you need. Focus deeply into your own eyes. See if the person in the mirror can silently fill in the blanks.

"The way I see myself holding back is ______."

"The way I see myself growing is ______."

7. After you have received an answer from the mirror move to a position standing before a trusted peer. The peer then rises and both group members look into each other's eyes and clasp hands. The client then shares: *"The way I am holding back is____. The way I am growing is____."*

8. The client and peer then thank each other and return to their seats.

9. After each client has participated, hold a discussion: Who did you see in the mirror? What feelings can you identify from your work? What was it like choosing a peer to open up to? What was it like being chosen?

Suggestions and pitfalls: This is intimate work. Clients should not be forced to stand before the mirror. Acknowledgment of resistance and the difficulty of truly looking at ourselves can be revealing in itself. Often it is helpful to have the counselor model the exercise before the clients begin their work. Quiet from the group when a client is doing the exercise helps endow the work with value.

HANDOUT #25

THE MAN IN THE GLASS

When you get what you want in your struggle for yourself
And the world makes you King for a day
Just go to a mirror and look at yourself
and see what that person has to say.

For it isn't your mother or father or wife
Whose judgment upon you must pass,
The person whose verdict counts most in your life
Is the one staring back from the glass.

Now, some people can call you a straight shootin' chum
and think you're a wonderful guy,
But the man in the glass says you're only a bum
If you won't look him straight in the eye.

He's the one to please, never mind all the rest
For he's with you clear up to the end,
And you've passed your most dangerous and difficult test
If the man in the glass can at least be your friend.

You can fool the whole world down the pathway of years
And get lots of pats on the back as you pass,
But your final reward will be heartaches and tears
If you cheat the man in the glass.

TOOLS OF SOBRIETY

Tools to get sober and stay sober are **actions**. Putting recovery into action not only ensures sobriety, it improves the quality of sobriety.

Individual Goal: To concretize and personalize the actions of sobriety. What are actions to get sober and stay sober? What tools are new to you? Which tools did you know, but forgot?

Group Goal: To bring the group together on the shared activity of brainstorming the actions of sobriety. Getting sober means not doing it alone. It is working together with other recovering people. And, it can be fun.

Materials needed: Blackboard, stopwatch, two separate brainstorming areas.

Presentation: The counselor explains the concept of a "tool." Cutting wood without an ax or a saw is an almost impossible task. It is just as difficult to get and remain sober without individual recovery tools.

In recovery, **Tools = Actions.**

For example: *"An AA meeting, in itself, is not a tool for sobriety if you do not attend it. The actions of getting up, leaving the house and participating at the meeting keep people sober."*

Staying sober is a combination of what you know and what you do. And, it means working together, sometimes under pressure. What are some pressures you are under?

This presentation uses the pressure of time constraint. It may be fun, even a bit silly. But, knowing and applying a tool for sobriety may save your life.

It is a game. The way you present the game will greatly affect the way it will be played. Some simple advice applies: Explain the game's structure and rules as clearly and simply as possible, and do it in a style that encourages participation, playfulness, and fun.

For example: *"We are going to play a game called Tools For Sobriety. You will be in two teams on either side of the room, but let me explain part of the game before we break into teams for both you, the contestants, and the television audience."*

If, as the leader, you are able to demonstrate the role playing with appropriate outrageous words and actions, you can serve as a model, encouraging all the players to quickly cast aside their inhibitions and join you. But watch out that you are not too silly for the group, or you might lose them rather than encourage them.

Warm-Up
Begin by a brief discussion of television game shows. If you were going to be on a television game show, which one would you choose? Which show has the best prizes?

Today we are going to actively brainstorm all the **Tools For Sobriety** we can think of. Some of you have some sober experience already, some of you have been in treatment before, and some of you have already demonstrated that you know how to stay away from a drink one day at a time.

A lecture on the Tools might be a bit boring. In order to make it more challenging we are going to use a game show format instead of a lecture.

It is one thing to be told what to do to stay sober and quite another to figure it out under pressure.

How To Play
This exercise is similar to the "Family Feud" television show. The counselor plays the host. The clients play the competing families.

Action:

1. Divide the group into two teams.

2. One member of each team is selected as a secretary to record the team's ideas and given writing materials.

3. Rearrange the chairs so that there are two rows facing each other. In a healthy family, no one person is any more or any less important than another. The same holds true for the participants of the two teams.

4. The teams are instructed to find a private area to:

   A. Invent a team name (5 points).

   B. Develop a list of tools for sobriety. What are you going to do to stay sober? (1 point for each tool.)

5. Challenging the other team's tool is allowed. **For example: A tool such as** "Ordering a soft drink at the bar" may be **challenged by the opposing team.** The client, then, will have one minute to justify the answer. The counselor/game show host serves as the judge.

6. Teams separate and are given ten minutes exactly to develop their lists of sobriety tools. At the end of ten minutes all pencils are down.

7. Teams regroup and the "television show" begins. The counselor/host introduces the show and uses the blackboard to record each team's points. A coin flip decides **which team will answer first.**

8. The list of tools is passed down the line and the two teams alternate answers. Both teams may have some similar tools of sobriety. Repetition of a tool between teams does not negate the answer as long as it can be shown that the action is on the brainstorm list.

9. The competition ends when one team exhausts their list.

10. The chairs are then rearranged to a **single group.** Brainstorming for additional tools with counselor input is the final stage of the action.

Suggestions: Applause and affirmations of quality tools can keep the game light and playful. Team lists and a list of the final brainstorm can be copied and given as a Handout.

HANDOUT #26

TOOLS

These tools are most easily accepted by group members when presented as a game:

1. AA Meetings (NA, CA, SLA, CODA, Al-Anon, etc.).
2. Sponsors.
3. Telephone treatment.
4. Get active — Central office, set up room, take a 12 Step position, i.e., coffee person.
5. Change old routines.
6. Change using friends.
7. HALT (hungry, angry, lonely, tired)
8. Remember the reality of last drink (avoiding euphoric recall).
9. Disease concept.
10. One day at a time.
11. Literature.
12. Step work.
13. New hobbies.
14. Exercise.
15. Avoid "pink cloud" syndrome.
16. Continued therapy.
17. Be aware of relapse symptoms/triggers.
18. Serenity Prayer.
19. Avoid the "if" traps.
20. Treat yourself to something nice.
21. No "Near Beer."
22. Slogans: "Think", "Easy Does It", "Live And Let Live."
23. "When all else fails . . . . follow directions."
24. Meditation.
25. Avoid adjunct addictions — food, sex, money, cigarettes, coffee, and/or a drug you have never abused before.
26. Alcohol/drug free home.
27. It's the first drink that gets you drunk.
28. Prayer.
29. Write a journal.
30. Make a recovery plan/contract.
31. Affirmations.
32. Identify with AA speakers, don't compare.
33. Help a newcomer.
34. Avoid using/drinking parties, get-togethers.
35. Use anger management tools — anger is the #1 relapse reason.
36. Practice assertive behavior.
37. Relaxation techniques.
38. Look at yourself in the mirror.
39. Eat something sweet — honey.
40. Art work.

UNFINISHED BUSINESS

While we are using alcohol or other drugs much gets left undone or unsaid. This exercise gives clients the opportunity to acknowledge the "holes" in our relationships.

Individual Goal: To practice our part in relating to others. To identify and experience the emotions of our past and present relationships.

Group Goal: Empathy and identification among group members is created as clients express themselves.

Presentation: Begin with a group discussion around the concept of unfinished business.

- What areas of your life did you ignore when you were using?
- What interests have been put aside?

All of us have 'unfinished business' with the people in our lives. **For example,** there may be some one you may have wished you had said something to, or done something with. Often chosen people include:

Someone who is very close to you.
Someone with whom you work.
Your children.
Someone with whom you had or have a communication problem.
Someone who died.
Someone from your childhood.
Your higher power.
Yourself.

Advise the group to take a moment to go inside themselves and think about who they might picture. **What has been left unsaid?** Place a chair in the front of the room. Ask the clients to pretend that there is someone in the chair with whom they have unfinished business. One at a time, invite them to address the person in the chair.

The counselor can facilitate the action of the group by modeling the exercise before asking for volunteers. We have so much unfinished business with the people in our lives and it is sometimes tempting to wish to address huge issues. This is not always necessary to do at first. Filling in the holes in our hearts and repairing our relationships often begins at the edges and with small actions. Please give an example.

Here's how it might look:

1. Suppose your client, Alice, has unfinished business with her deceased mother. Alice informs the group that her mother is in the empty chair and Alice tells her mother her "unfinished business".

2. Should Alice ask her mother in the chair a question, direct Alice to assume the role of her mother. Alice moves to the empty chair.

3. The counselor then assumes the role of the client, Alice. Repeat the question to Alice who has become her mother. This will give Alice the opportunity to answer from the point of view of her mother. After "mother" responds, direct Alice to resume her own role and stand facing the empty chair once more, to continue her "unfinished business".

After each client has been given the opportunity to work, hold a group discussion.

What feelings came up for you?
What resistance did you have?
What unfinished business do you still carry?

ANGER

Anger is a key issue in recovery. Many of us respond to certain situations with blame, rage, resentment, guilt and even physical abuse as a result of repressed anger. Many of us have learned to avoid any expression that even remotely suggests anger in order to "Keep the Peace". This presentation explores the many faces of anger and gives methods of dealing with anger which clients can use to bring more comfort and emotional balance to their lives.

Individual Goal: Clients will understand their anger and ways to deal with it.

Group Goal: Group cohesion and communication improve as clients share feelings, experiences, and develop a common understanding of anger, anger triggers, and resentment.

Materials needed: Blackboard, Handouts — "Risk," and "So What Can I Do About My Anger?"

One of the most important issues for people in recovery is anger. Understanding what it is, what it looks like, and what to do about it can keep people sober.

Let's use the slogan "Keep It Simple". Very simply, what is anger?

Anger is a feeling. One complication that many people add is to make value judgments around feelings. **Example:** *"But I shouldn't be angry." "Why should I get angry? It won't do any good."* These are ways of saying anger is bad. A feeling is neither good nor bad. "Shoulds" or "shouldn'ts" have nothing to do with our feelings. **Feelings simply are.**

Perhaps because there are value judgments around anger we call the feeling of anger many different names. **Example:** Someone may furiously say, *"I am not angry! I am not angry! I am just very upset!"* Indeed, anger comes in many different shapes and colors.

Ask for a volunteer to come before the group to model anger. If you could not use the word "anger" to describe what it looks like Jim is feeling, what words would you use?

Brainstorm with the group to determine the descriptions we often give anger.

Create a list on the blackboard.

Anger is often called:

pissed-off
nasty
chip on the shoulder
mean
attitude
frustrated
snobby
envious
suspicious
upset
anxious
intolerant
cold
distrustful
hate-filled
tense
jealous
sarcastic
cynical
resentful, etc.

Sometimes we use these words to more clearly define our anger. At other times, we use these words to deny our anger. In recovery, we hear a lot about denial. It has no place in recovery. In sobriety, we express our feelings, not to change other people and certainly not to purposely hurt them, but to share with them who we are, how we feel.

Expressing anger and letting people know who we are is very risky proposition. It can be very scary. Here is a short poem about risk.

"Risk" — Handout #27

Ask for a volunteer to "risk" reading it aloud.

HANDOUT #27

RISK

To laugh is to risk appearing a fool

To weep is to risk appearing sentimental.

To reach out for another is to risk
involvement

To expose feelings is to risk rejection

To place your dreams before the crowd is to
risk ridicule

To love is to risk not being loved in return

To go forward in the face of overwhelming odds
is to risk failure

But risks must be taken because the greatest
hazard in life is to risk nothing.

The person who risks nothing does nothing,
has nothing, is nothing.

He may avoid suffering and sorrow,

But he cannot learn, feel, change, grow, or love.

Chained by his certitude's, he is a slave.

He has forfeited his freedom.

Only a person who takes risks is free.

Anonymous

Have you ever felt trapped by your anger? To take the risk to express anger can be frightening. What are some fears you may have in expressing anger? Brainstorm with the group. Make a list on the blackboard.

Fears about expressing anger :

Fear of rejection.
Fear of losing control.
Fear of being counter-attacked.
Fear of hurting others.
Fear of feeling guilty afterwards.
Fear that anger is not acceptable to others.
Fear that others will see an expression of anger as a weakness.

Many times, fear and anger are intertwined. How do you know when you are feeling anger? What are the physical symptoms of anger? Brainstorm with the group.

Physical symptoms of anger:

headaches
hot in the face
vision changes (either focused or diffused)
tension
energy increase
hyperventilation
rapid heart beat
clenched jaw, etc.

Notice how the feelings of anger are similar to the feelings of fear. Asking ourselves, **"How do I feel, right now?"** can help us become more aware of how subtle our feelings can be. Learning how to identify which feeling we're really experiencing gives us more clarity about the solutions.

It is an interesting phenomenon that men and women often react differently to feelings of anger. In our society, men seem to get positive reinforcement for expressing anger and women do not. Angry men are often seen as strong and powerful. A women who expresses anger is called "a bitch."

In getting clear about the difference between anger and fear for both men and women, it is important to ask, **"What's underneath this feeling?"** Many times men will find fear under the anger. Of course, these are generalities. Just as feelings are not good or bad, neither do they have gender. Anger and fear are part of human emotion for everyone.

Two important questions to ask are:

What feeling is underneath this behavior?

How do I feel, right now?

One theory about anger is that "Anger turned inward is depression." Do you agree with this idea?

People "bottle" anger, "stuff" anger, and "hide" anger. This can be a conscious choice or a learned way of behaving, ingrained from our early childhood. Brainstorm with the group.

What are the signs of hidden anger?

Signs of hidden anger :

- clenched jaw
- insomnia
- over-sleeping
- loss of appetite
- over-eating
- smiling all the time
- tension in shoulders and neck
- anxiety
- passive/aggressive behavior toward others
- procrastination
- being late
- worrying
- sighing
- chain smoking
- foot tapping
- being chronically tired
- mumbling under your breath
- going over and over the situation in your mind, etc.

Hidden anger is sometimes called cold anger. **Cold anger, resentment, has been identified as the #1 reason for relapse.**

Anger can come in a flash. As fast as a bullet. This type of anger is called a **trigger**. Looking at your triggers is best done when you're in good space, when you are relatively comfortable and willing to be aware of anger. **Identifying triggers** will make it easier to express your anger when the situation happens.

Let us take a moment to inventory your specific anger triggers. The counselor writes at the top of the board:

TRIGGERS

I get angry when . . . .

Some of these situations may be big while others may be small and quirky, specific only to you. All of them are okay. **Example:** (Model one of your own triggers) *"I get angry when I step in gum on the sidewalk."*

Brainstorm with the group and quickly fill the board. (For specific work with triggers, see the group "The Missing Link.")

Some of the anger on the board seems justified. There are some terrible situations listed. As people in recovery, we must always be on the lookout for **justifying** our anger. **Example:** *"I have every right to be angry." "I am right and you are wrong!"*

This is called self-righteous behavior. It is a dubious luxury and can drive us back to old, sick behaviors. **Example:** *"I'm right. I'm right. I'm right."*

With **self-righteous anger** comes blaming, pouting, criticizing, accusing, and judging. These are the **behaviors that lead us to relapse. Example:** Suppose two people were really, truly rude to me at an AA meeting. They took my seat when I went to the restroom. They jostled me and spilled my coffee. Not only did they not apologize, they laughed and looked at me with a condescending glance.

I might have every right in the world to feel angry. Indulging my self-righteous anger would not help me, however. Stewing and brooding about their behavior would keep me from benefiting from the other eighteen people in the room. *If I never returned to the AA meeting, I would be the one losing out.* **Self-righteous anger can never work for us.**

From the list, it is obvious that everyone here can understand what it is like to feel angry or irritated. Many of you experience anger at similar issues. Not everyone's triggers are the same or of the same intensity. It is important to know that:

Anger is about me. It is my feeling and only I am responsible for it !!

People often say, *"You make me angry."* or *"This situation makes me very angry."* It is built into our language and into our thinking. In sobriety, ***"I am responsible for my feelings."***

I do not blame.
I do not blame others for my feelings.
I do not blame situations for my feelings.

This is a difficult concept. Here is a brief example that helps me realize that my anger is about me and my process. I call it the **$50 million lottery game**.

> **Angrily state:** *"It makes me angry to step on old chewing gum on the sidewalk. Inconsiderate slobs who have no consideration for others make me furious. They ought to be shot. Or, at the very least, made to clean the sidewalks. With a toothbrush! I'm so angry, I could kill! "*
>
> Now, I win the $50 million lottery. I step in the same chewing gum.
>
> **Happily state:** *"Oh, look I've stepped on gum. Must be God's way of telling me I need new shoes. I think I'll go buy a pair. A pair?!? I'll go buy 10 pairs! This is the last time I will ever walk down this street. Next time, I'll be driving my new car. These poor sidewalks are filthy. Maybe I'll donate a sidewalk cleaner to the city. Nothing can stop me now!"*

Of course, this is an absurd example. I do not have 50 million dollars. But, my anger is not about the outside situation. It is not really about the gum on the sidewalk. **<u>It is about me</u>**. Hopefully, this game can help you realize **your** anger is about **<u>you</u>**. Where **<u>you</u>** are coming from. What **<u>your</u>** triggers are.

So, what can you do about your anger? This Handout is only a beginning. Go over the "So What Can I Do About My Anger?" Handout # 28. Take time to discuss each point. Ask the group if they have additional suggestions.

Notes To Clinicians: About Rage

It is important to assist the client to understand that there is a world of difference between the feelings of anger and those of rage. The two are not the same nor do they derive from the same source.

This anger group is extremely useful for working with **anger.** It will compound the frustration of a client who is attempting to "handle" **rage.** Explain to a client who suffers from rage that usually anger is a response to one of two things: perceived injustice, or the inability to control. Like a wave on the ocean, anger has a beginning, a crescendo and an end.

Rage is a reaction to repressed feelings of helplessness and hopelessness. The helplessness is not experienced by the individual. To avoid feeling helpless as a child, the feeling is sublimated and attached to one which has power - rage. Imagine walking along and stepping on a land mine. **Rage** is experienced as a **sudden explosion**. It is an internal explosion with the same loss of control as a land mine. It helps to explain to people who have rage that they have internal emotional charges which are like depth charges deep in the ocean.

Treating rage like anger is harmful to the client. In treatment, they can develop a plan or "fire drill" for their rage until they are able to work with a skilled clinician who can walk with them through their repressed helplessness from childhood abuse.

HANDOUT #28

SO WHAT CAN I DO ABOUT MY ANGER?

1. **Apply Step One.** "We admitted we were powerless over our anger and that our lives had become unmanageable." By simply admitting we are powerless to control what, where, and when we feel angry, we deepen our awareness of the very nature of feelings. We have no more control over any feeling — mad, glad, sad, or bad—than we do over thoughts that pop in an out of our minds.

2. Remember that **anger is a feeling**. Everyone feels it. Anger is natural, healthy, non-evil, and human. It moves us to resolve conflicts.

3. Feeling anger and acting out anger are not the same thing, therefore, **I am responsible for what I do**.

4. **My anger is my own.** The other person did not "make" me angry.

5. **Get to know your anger triggers.** "Find your own buttons, so you'll know when they're pushed."

6. **Don't set yourself up to get angry.** If your temperature rises when you are waiting in a slow line at the super market, shop at a less busy time of day. Work at finding resolutions.

7. **Talk about your feelings.** Friends, sponsors, other group members, and family can often support **you** and your feelings. Do **not** use them to make yourself "right".

8. **Avoid justifying your anger.** Remember, self-righteous anger is a killer.

9. **State your feelings directly**, with appropriate non-verbal cues. For example: "*I feel angry when you . . . .*" If you are genuinely angry, a smile is inappropriate.

10. **Develop coping strategies** to deal with the discomfort of anger. For Example: Relaxation, physical exercise, breathing, taking "time outs", affirmations.

11. **Practice assertively expressing your anger.** Avoid name-calling, put-downs, one-upmanship.

12. **Pray.** The Serenity Prayer helps with both external resolution and internal resolution.

13. **Deal with issues as they arise.** Avoid stewing about an issue for hours, days, or weeks. If you are unable to address the conflict immediately, arrange a specific time when you can and will.

14. **Work toward resolution.** Resolution of the conflict. Resolution of the feeling.

THE MISSING LINK

INTRODUCTION:

Many of our clients have difficulty with impulse control. Some are greatly affected by emotional "triggers." Both of these situations are experienced by clients as a feeling followed by an action or behavior.

Example: "I was angry so I hit him," or:

My feeling —— **leads to** ——> **my behavior.**

As a result of this perceived dynamic, individuals frequently feel powerless over their behavior and powerless over their actions.

The actual experiential dynamic is more like this:

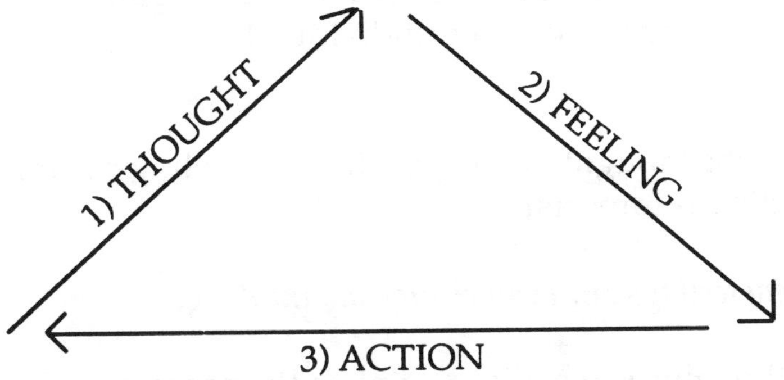

For reasons not obvious to the client, they have repressed the **"thought"** from their conscious awareness.

Example: *"I thought I was in danger, I was angry so I hit him."*

Identification of the thought is the **"missing link"** to understanding why they have specific automatic responses to particular feelings and situations.

To break the addiction cycle and avoid relapse, the client needs to become aware of his repressed thoughts. It is these thoughts which lead to emotional triggers and ensuing behaviors which ultimately lead to relapse.

OBJECTIVES:

1. To allow the client to identify the link between thoughts, feelings, and behavior.

2. To recognize the impact of behavior in either reinforcing recovery or moving one toward relapse.

3. To identify the feelings to which the client attaches values.

Materials needed: Blackboard

Group set-up: Have the group sit in a semicircle facing the blackboard.

Opening Statement:

In this group, our goal is to explore the link between thoughts, feelings, and behavior. "Our behavior is the external manifestation of what I think in response to what I feel."

I THINK ⟶ I FEEL ⟶ I ACT.

In order to understand this process and use it in recovery, we must be clear on all three steps of this process and how they work for us, individually.

1. We must identify the thoughts we have when the feeling occurs. To learn to separate thinking and feeling is important.

   I cannot change my feelings but I can change my thinking.

   Identifying the thoughts is the missing link in the process, and the most difficult part to see and understand. Our tendency can be to automatically or ***unconsciously combine*** **the feeling and the thought together. Over time, we are unable to separate the two.**

The thought can sometimes be a value or belief about the feeling.

For example: Most of us grew up in environments where we were taught that certain feelings were not acceptable and not okay. Our parents (teachers) taught us what they had learned about feelings from their parents. If I grew up in a home where expressing anger was considered "bad" behavior, I might have been spanked or grounded when I got mad and told someone about it. **I would have learned that anger is bad.** *As an adult, when I feel the emotion "**anger**," I attach the thought "**anger is bad**."*

The judgment that "anger is bad", **is connected to the thought, not the feeling.** However, I cannot make this distinction so I conclude that the feeling "anger" itself is bad. My behavior will reflect this belief:

When I am angry, I will act "bad" automatically. Perhaps, I will become violent and throw things or automatically try to hide my anger so no one will know. The fact is that anger has **no value unless I give it value.** I can change my mind about what it means to me. If I do this, *my behavior when I am angry can be different.*

2. We must learn to identify our feelings.

We have already made considerable progress in this area. We have been practicing naming and clarifying feelings such as: anger, shame, guilt, peacefulness, and contentment. We have also had experience in sharing these feelings with others.

3. We must identify how our behavior is connected to our thoughts.

We are always responsible for our own behavior in recovery. A big part of sobriety is owning up to what we do or do not do.

Remember:

IF I ALWAYS DO WHAT I ALWAYS DID, I ALWAYS GET WHAT I ALWAYS GOT!

We have made many changes in behavior already. Since we can see our behavior most clearly, behavior is a good place to begin the changing.

This is the process we are going to explore:

On the blackboard, make three columns labeled **Thought, Emotion, Behavior.**

1. Ask the group to generate a feelings list.

2. When the list is completed, ask group members to identify the values ("good, bad") which they have learned about these feelings. This is not a time for group therapy so just acknowledge contributions with "great" or "that's a good one," then move on.

3. Ask the group which feeling they would like to explore in greater detail. The most common choices are: Anger, shame, and sadness. If the group cannot decide or they decide to be passive, then you choose. "Anger" will get their energy going **and is the example we have selected below.**
Write the feeling in the Feeling Column below.

4. Next, ask members to consider a situation in which the feeling occurred. Have them describe the situation in one sentence.

   Example: "My boss yelled at me for something I didn't do." Then, ask them to tell the group a **thought** they had when this event took place. *Write this in the Thought column.*

5. Go to the Behavior column and ask the client what he did. *Enter the behavior on the list.* Be sure to instruct the group to keep it simple and give examples to assure answers are short and specific.

6. Lastly, have the group review the behavior list and consider whether the behavior described is more likely to lead to recovery or relapse. Next to the behavior list,
   place a **"D"** for disease or relapse behavior, or
   place an **"R"** for recovery behavior.

Sample:

"My boss yelled at me for something I didn't do."

THOUGHT	FEELING	BEHAVIOR	
"That's a lie."	ANGER	D	"I called him a liar."
"How dare you."		D	"I called him a liar and walked out."
"It's all your fault."		D	"I ignored him."
"Would you explain more?"		R	"I asked her to explain."
"All you do is complain."		D	"I went out and got drunk."

If you have time remaining, you may continue the group using the same behavior column to help clients identify what defense mechanisms are associated with those behaviors marked "D".

Example:

Behavior	Defense Mechanism
I punched him out.	HOSTILITY
I went out and got drunk.	BLAME

The group may also brainstorm about recovery tools and options to replace the "old behaviors and thinking."

GRIEF AND LOSS

Objectives:

1. Clients will learn and identify the stages of grief related to chemical dependency.

2. Clients will verbalize where they see themselves in the grief process, giving specific examples related to their stages.

3. Clients will identify their specific losses associated with alcoholism/addiction.

Materials needed: Blackboard

This material is covered in two parts.

Part I includes: Group Loss List and Lecture on the process and stages of grief.

Part II includes: Individual Client Review of his/her grief process.

Opening Statement:

All of us have experienced losses as a result of our alcoholism. Today, we will be looking at those losses and discussing the process of healing. Facing our powerlessness over drugs and alcohol is the first step in our recovery.

1. Generate a list on the blackboard of losses the group members have experienced as a result of their addiction. Identify losses in these areas: Physical and emotional health, finances, relationships, legal status, self-esteem, etc. Also find out some group totals - the total number of cars wrecked by the group, total finances, and so on. (See last page in this section for examples.)

2. Lecture: Main points are in bold print.

Definition of Grief:

Grief is a normal reaction and process associated with anticipated or actual loss. It is a universal experience. Loss, great or small is always accompanied by grief. Emotional pain is a part of this process. As we walk through the stages of healing, the pain lessens and we come to accept the realities of our loss. Let us explore these stages.

These stages of grief were identified by Dr. Elizabeth Kubler Ross in her work with dying cancer patients. They apply to any disease process. We'll be discussing them in relationship to the disease of chemical dependency. **(Review them on the blackboard.)**

Denial:

Denial is a psychological avoidance of reality.

In the normal and successful process of grieving, denial is temporary. Often the loss causes a "shock effect."

> **For example:** "No, this can't be true. No way I'm alcoholic." or "It's not possible."

Being diagnosed as an alcoholic means that there are tough realities to face. As with cancer, it is not easy to believe that we have a chronic, progressive, terminal disease that affects every area of our lives and requires major lifestyle changes. Denial occurs.

Denial is the natural first step of recovery. However, prolonged denial for the alcoholic leads to greater and greater loss in health, relationships, possessions, self-esteem, etc.

Anger:

When we work through the denial and face the reality of having the disease of chemical dependency, it is normal to be angry about it.

> **For example:** "How could this happen to me? It's not fair! I like alcohol!"

In our powerlessness, we may look for a place or person who caused the loss. **For example:** We may blame God, or fate, society, or our family for our predicament. The way in which we experience or express our anger can work for or against us in this process.

In its healthy form, an expression of anger is energizing, and it can give us the impetus to move into positive action. In its destructive form, this anger can build bitter resentments, or find its outlet in verbal or emotional abuse toward others.

In this stage, we experience rebellion. We need to acknowledge our anger and express it.

Bargaining:

In the bargaining stage we do not deny the disease but tend to minimize the extent and impact it has on our lives. We do this by resisting making all of the necessary changes

required to fully recover. In dealing with our alcoholism, we attempt to regain a sense of control.

We bargain for ways to deal with our disease without making the necessary major changes in our life styles. We bargain about what we need to do to stay sober. The fact is, it cannot be done. I cannot recover and "be the same old me." Recovery requires a major change. We try to find **"the easier softer way,"** and use **"half-measures"** to remedy our using and drinking.

> **For example:** *"I can just quit drinking and everything else will work out."* We begin trying to cut deals with God. *"I'll quit using if you give me my wife back."*

This stage is also a normal part of the grief process. Remaining in this stage too long, however, can be devastating to the alcoholic and place us at high risk for relapse.

Depression:

In the depression stage, we feel the sorrow and pain of our disease.

Pain hurts! In our alcoholism, all of us have used chemicals and alcohol to help us avoid feeling pain. With feelings of sorrow also comes intense loneliness and feelings of helplessness. Our drugs and booze have served as our greatest comfort in dealing with pain. *"How can I get through without them!"* Being willing to feel the pain of being chemically dependent is not at all easy. It means taking a big risk and allowing ourselves to be vulnerable. When we are in pain, it can feel like it will never end.

In the depression stage, *we feel the pain of the reality of losing our ability to ever be "normal" again. We also experience the loss of our best friend, alcohol and drugs.* Some of us even have thoughts of suicide. All of these feelings are real.

We have faced much tragedy and loss in having this disease. We need to experience its pain in order to find healing. If we allow ourselves this process, our pain will diminish and move us on to the next stage, acceptance.

Acceptance:

Acceptance is the final stage and the goal of the grieving process.

I am powerless over being alcoholic and the devastation it has caused in my life." Having mourned all of this, we can now proceed with our lives. The resistance has vanished. We are ready to go to any length to address our alcoholism. We finally understand that sobriety is our priority. We experience calm and tranquillity. Life has new meaning and we embrace our new path.

The grief process does not take us on a straight path. We can move in and out of these stages and be in several or all of the stages at once.

For example: A person can be in the anger and bargaining stages simultaneously.

Examples of the stages of grief are:

Denial: *"I noticed that I questioned myself today about whether or not I'm really an alcoholic."*

Anger: *"I'm angry about all the time that I wasted, especially flunking out of school."*

Bargaining: *"I still feel I can hang around with using friends and not use myself. I don't think that I need to go to a meeting every day."*

Depression: *"I've been crying every night. I feel discouraged and sad."*

Acceptance: *"It doesn't bother me to work a program if I want to stay sober."*

List all of these stages on the board.

With the remaining time of the group, each client will come up individually to the blackboard.

First, they will place their initials next to the stages that they presently fit into.

Then, they will go back to the stages that they have marked and explain to the group exactly how and why they are in that stage by giving an example.

When each person is finished, have them ask the group for feedback. Does the group agree or disagree with the stage the client is in? What do they see and how do they see it? Direct the feedback to be simple and direct without advice giving or judgment. All of the stages are healthy.

This process takes time and hard work. The more willing we are to go through it, the quicker we will benefit. Avoiding this process is dangerous for alcoholics. We soon move into our old ways of coping and the relapse process replaces the grieving process. Make your choice!

HANDOUT # 29

"THERE IS NO BIRTH OF CONSCIOUSNESS WITHOUT PAIN"
C. Jung

GRIEF STAGES:

Denial
Anger
Bargaining
Depression
Acceptance

LOSSES:

Self Respect
Jobs
Relationships
Marriages
Children
Self-Love
Money
Houses
Spirituality
Sensitivity
Education
Friendships
Emotional Stability
Pride
Honesty
Alcohol
Control
Ability to Communicate
Respect from Others
Ability to Think Clearly

SUFFERING

The following story best describes the essence of this group:

An elderly couple had recently lost their only child. They were devastated and their hearts completely broken. Why had she died so young? How could God explain this? How would they live without her?

They searched for these answers with each other, with their friends, and in their prayers. They found no answers. They finally went to an old woman who was known for her wisdom and compassion. With tears in their eyes, they begged her to reveal how they could relieve themselves of their endless and horrible suffering. She touched them gently and replied, *"I am unable to remove your pain. I can only teach you how to make it sacred."*

Our clients have suffered. Some needlessly, some self-inflicted, and some incomprehensibly in ways we cannot imagine. As a society, we abhor pain, and we shun the darkness. We demonstrate this by our use of "fix it" pills, one-step therapies, and "cute" shaming and judgmental messages like "suffering is mandatory, misery is optional," as if we had experienced and known this pain ourselves. We shun the darkness and the pain, in ourselves and for others.

From our darkness and suffering begins our healing. Seeds cannot grow unless they are planted underground. Babies are created and grow in the darkness of our womb. From the depths of our suffering blossoms compassion. *Our pain gives depth as feeling beings. To be shut off from our pain is to suffocate that part of us that grows from having suffered. To be able to give meaning to our pain makes us and our pain sacred.*

This is a very simple group and, if done well, can absolutely transform your clients and your group.

Your introduction is the essential ingredient in making this a magical group. You need to create an emotional space for your clients to show you their pain.

Soften the lights and inform the group about the emotional vulnerability they will be asked to share, some for the first time ever.

Ask them if they can leave their judgment, advice giving, and "fix it" responses outside of the group room.

This group is not about fixing anything. It is about **being**, exposing the darkness, and letting it be silent. *The silence has her own voice and she will provide a message about the healing which is growing from the suffering.*

Ask each group member to identify two ways or examples of their suffering. Let the first example be superficial.

Ask them to find a second, deeper example.

Put them both on the chalkboard. Placing examples on the chalkboard keeps them from being hidden again.

Read, or have somebody read the story at the beginning.

Inform the group that they are to imagine that they have a "guardian angel." What gift does the angel want to give them from their suffering?

So, if the example is — *"I lost my son,"* the gift might be, *"I understand the pain of other fathers."* Reframe this in a way that might be more universal. *"Are you saying that you have developed compassion?"* If this is not correct for them then suggest another gift. If it is correct, ask them how they have seen this gift already in their lives — *"How have you become more compassionate?"* After they have been given a moment to experience this example, move on to their second, deeper example.

Leave it there, do not explore therapy issues or let a group member pull them out of that emotional space by "making them happy."

When each member has had their turn, ask the group if they can discuss the meaning and role of suffering.

Let them each relate their understanding of its purpose.

Remind them that endless suffering is about blocking ourselves from the gift underneath it, so a part of suffering is to be able to let go of the pain and suffering, and move into acceptance.

Some suggestions to keep the group going are that pain:

1. *Gives us compassion* — We understand other's pain and it links us together.

2. *Shows us what is beautiful and precious in life* — We can appreciate life and love more fully.

3. *Tell us what is important in our lives* — The workaholic parent who loses one child suddenly makes time for the other children.

4. *Gives us new strength* — Those of us who have survived some kind of torture, abuse or tragedy, have a different type of strength than those of us who have not.

5. *Opens us up* — For those of us who choose to deal with our pain, we are forced to find the meaning or purpose to our life.

6. *Defines us* — I am the kind of person who can accept tragedy and still find the space to love.

Close the group by bringing everybody "in." Some people took more risks than others and feel vulnerable or isolated.

Have the group stand and join hands.

Ask them to look around the group for one minute, acknowledging silently each person and their contribution.

Thank the group for providing safety and honoring each other.

This group requires some follow-up. If you cannot do it that day, establish the date and time it will be done.

Check in with members about what came up for them:

- Did they trigger any emotional land mines?
- How are they handling it?
- What changed for them?
- How did this group affect the way they see themselves and their lives with respect to their spirituality and recovery?

HANDOUT #30

SUFFERING

An elderly couple had recently lost their only child. They were devastated and their hearts completely broken. Why had she died so young? How could God explain this? How would they live without her?

They searched for these answers with each other, with their friends, and in their prayers. They found no answers. They finally went to an old woman who was known for her wisdom and compassion. With tears in their eyes, they begged her to reveal how they could relieve themselves of their endless and horrible suffering. She touched them gently and replied, *"I am unable to remove your pain. I can only teach you how to make it sacred."*

SPIRITUALITY

The process of healing from the disease of chemical dependency includes healing **physically, emotionally,** and **spiritually.** In our disease, we lose sight of who we truly are. As we slide deeper and deeper into our addictions, we develop irrational beliefs, delusions, and faulty perceptions of ourselves and others. Life's meaning and purpose escape us. **We become unaware of our real reason for being.**

Spiritual recovery is a difficult concept for many to grasp because we've had so many preconceived notions about it. While the idea of spirituality seems inaccessible for many of us in early recovery, *our recovery itself is dependent upon it.* The principals of spirituality are so simple that most of us miss them.

The path of spiritual recovery leads us to our true selves. Our "True Self" remains inside of us. It has been buried under years of addiction and a lifetime of lies. Spiritual recovery reunites us with ourselves.

Our process of spiritual healing begins the moment we decide to work toward our recovery.

Consider this story:

Michelangelo was preparing to do a sculpture. In front of him was the stone he would use. He carefully contemplated the stone and began to chisel. When his work was finished he had created the Madonna and Child. A friend asked him, *"How did you create such a beautiful statue?"* Michelangelo answered, *"I saw the Madonna and Child in the stone and simply chiseled away that part of stone which did not belong".*

How many of you when sober have looked back at your using and said, *"That was not the real me?"* You understood this. The real you lies in the midst of your own piece of stone.

Spiritual recovery is the chiseling away of all of those pieces that don't belong to us.

The chisel is in the hands of the "sculptor" (our Higher Power).

Our tools are honesty, openness, and willingness.

> **Honesty** refers to our seeing and acknowledging truth.
>
> **Openness** gives us the ability to learn and dissolves our self imposed limitations.
>
> **Willingness** is the key to change and positive action.

We use these tools to direct us to the "sculptor", whoever, and whatever that may be. We trust that the sculptor will reveal "The Madonna" in our stone.

SPIRITUAL AWAKENING

For some of us this is a vague or religious concept. We might envision ourselves engulfed in light, knocked off our horse by lightening, or being visited by an angel. For most of us, though, it is a gradual **wakening up.** In recovery the process is simple and the results are the "miracle".

Let us look at how each of these spiritual principals works.

1. Honesty :
We have a disease that is characterized by denial which shields us from the truth. How then can we see or come to know the truth? We feel it in our "spirit. "Our truth is there, it just needs to be uncovered. Here is a simple test for checking out the truth"

> **A. Place the diagram below on the board.**
> Thought (Head)
> Feeling (Heart)
> Knowing (Gut)

First, I **think** the truth. We know as alcoholics that our thinking is not necessarily reliable. We check it out with a sponsor. We move the thought to our hearts, and there, we consider whether this honestly "feels like the truth". If so, we move on to the **"feeling"** of truth or to our gut (lower abdomen) and ask: "Do I know this to be the truth?" If you have accessed the truth it will be clear to you **by the feeling.** If you experience doubt or confusion, it is an indication that you're off the path.

2. Openness :
Openness refers to the process of *"letting go "of old ideas and beliefs.* It means becoming teachable, **to seek knowledge and understanding.** It is a kind of ongoing exploration. We have been taught that learning ends when we find the answer, and that the answer is final and absolute. This is another false assumption. In fact, when *we assume to have an answer, then our ability to learn ceases.* To be teachable in recovery means that we must throw away the answers. To develop spirituality means that we know is there is infinite knowledge and limitless truth.

3. Willingness :
Willingness is the process of readiness to act. Identifying the truth and being opened to new information are internal processes. Willingness to do something about it and **putting it into action** makes it real on the outside.

God can't make a Stradivarius violin without Stradivarius.

4. The Twelve Steps:
The Twelve Steps are our guide to a spiritual awakening. A *spiritual awakening simply means that one's spirit is awake.* Using the spiritual principles of honesty, openness, and willingness, we work the Steps in the order they are written. If we are honest and thorough in all of the Steps, we will become spiritually awake. ***"Having had a spiritual awakening** as the result of these Steps, we tried to carry this message to alcoholics and to practice these principles in all our affairs".*

Group Discussion:

1. What is spirituality to you?

2. What is your spirit and how do you know if you're in touch with it?

3. How do you practice your spirituality?

   Example: Prayer and meditation, walks in nature.

4. Do you have any "old ideas" about spirituality that block you in pursuing your connection to your spirit?

   Example: Concept of a punishing God.

5. What are some spiritual principles?

   Example: humility, acceptance, forgiveness.

6. How have you begun to apply the principles of honesty, openness, and willingness in your life?

7. Can you allow others the freedom to experience their spirituality differently than you do?

Remember that spiritual growth is a process.

It takes time.

If we hang in there, we will find our Madonna in the Stone!

TO CHANGE OR NOT TO CHANGE

Recovery requires change, change, and more change. This is a difficult and threatening task for alcoholics. Change to what? How am I supposed to do this? For many of us, changing will not feel natural or comfortable.

Many of us are like the horse called the "barn rat". This horse is so emotionally attached to the barn that when the rider points him off in any other direction, he walks slower and slower. When he's turned back towards the barn, he joyously races back in.

The "barn rat" is not wild about change. Neither are we.

This group will allow the "barn rats" to be comfortable with their new direction as they will now be familiar with it. Hopefully, when sprung loose, they will race into their recovery barn.

This exercise is a fun and empowering experience. In a non-threatening way, it gives your clients an opportunity to really see the need to change their using behaviors and attitudes by acting them out. It empowers your client by allowing them to identify and practice recovering behaviors without the implied threat that in order to recover, they need to somehow magically transform into saints overnight.

Materials: Blackboard, sheet of paper, assigned secretary, a coin

Explain to the group that it is easy to tell when somebody's in their disease or in recovery. Whether they are drinking or not, their behaviors and attitudes demonstrate this.

For example:

> A person who only quits drinking/using but changes nothing else is considered a **dry drunk**. They have not worked through any of their denial and remain self-centered and self-willed.
>
> The person in **recovery** is also easy to spot as they are more honest, open, and willing. They are better listeners, are non-judgmental, and accept the challenges of life as they come.

This group is about letting people see that they have a choice about being a dry drunk or in recovery. The only way to do this is to do both!

Using the blackboard, write a list of behaviors.
Set up two columns, **A & B,** next to those behaviors.
Column A reads: My disease, The Old Me, A Dry Drunk.
Column B reads: My Recovery, Who I Can Be, Recovering.

The board looks like this:

BEHAVIORS:	A. MY DISEASE: THE OLD ME A DRY DRUNK (List of Behaviors)	B. MY RECOVERY: WHO CAN I BE RECOVERING (List of Behaviors)
Honesty list a few →	ex: I lie to my wife about my using	ex: honest to my wife about my using
Attitude		
Anger		
Responsibility		
Participation in AA & Treatment		
Relationships		
Spirituality		
Denial		

Delete or choose other behaviors as appropriate for your group.

Have Client #1 choose a secretary; Client #2.

Ask Client #1 to go down through **the list of behaviors.** Chart their responses on the chalkboard. Ask the secretary to copy it down on a sheet of paper.

Using honesty as the first example, ask Client # 1 to now respond to Column A. **How is their** honesty affected **when they are in their disease?** How does that look to others — how do we see this?

> **Example:** *"I lie."* **More specifically,** *"I lie to my wife about my using."*

How is their honesty affected **when they are in recovery?** How do we see that?

> **Example:** *"I am honest."* **More specifically,** *"I do not lie to my wife about my using."*

Continue this list until it is complete, then hand Client #1 their sheet of behaviors and move on to the next client.

Note: Make certain that they list specific behaviors **that are measurable.** If they say something vague like *"I'll feel happy,"* respond with, *"So, I'll see you **smiling**"* (a measurable behavior).

When the group is finished, instruct them that being in recovery or in their disease **is a choice.** Most people won't take a job unless they have found out what the job is about, met the boss, discussed salaries, etc. Has anybody ever signed up for the military and six weeks later said, *"Oh, my God!"*?

The goal here is to be familiar with being in their disease barn, or in their recovery barn, so they have the power to make a choice later.

Ask Client #1 to choose somebody to flip a coin for them.

> **Heads** — They are in recovery for four hours. They act out all their recovery behaviors no matter what.
>
> **Tails** — They are in their disease for four hours. No matter what is going on, they act out in their disease. Period.

So, the coin says that they're **"in recovery"** today and their wife burns the dinner or the AA speaker is an obnoxious egomaniac, they have to compliment and hug their wife, speak in AA and thank the speaker!

If they are **"in their disease"** and their wife made their favorite meal and they loved the AA speaker, they have to criticize their wife and find fault with the speaker and AA, and complain miserably to somebody.

They must obey the coin. Variations may include the amount of time they act out these behaviors.

Follow-up Process Group:

This is not about you or the group trying to change your clients! This group is only empowering if your clients can make their own decisions to change no matter how insignificant or absurd the change might seem.

Ask them: (See Scaling Technique)

- Which role was more difficult for you?
- Which day seemed better to you?
- On a scale of 1 to 10 — 1, being horrible and 10, being spectacular — how was being in your disease?
- How was it being in recovery?
- **What seemed to make the difference?**

Reframe the behavior **that made the difference** in a way which implies that they could **benefit by increasing that behavior,** (accent the positive).

So, if the difference to feeling better was that they did not lie, a reframe might be, *"So, not lying for four hours seemed to change your day, and you felt like a 6 on the scale. To go to a 7 on the scale, how many hours of honesty would you need? Five hours? That's pretty interesting . . . ."* (Do not suggest the changes for them!) If they do not come up with a solution to going to a 7, simply repeat your statement.

Remember to observe the changes that improved their subjective sense of feeling better and to repeat those behaviors back to them.

Every group has the passive or passive-aggressive client. They won't identify any positive behaviors which changed their days. **Simply paraphrase their negative statements:** *"You do not know why you had a 3 star day in your disease and a 5 star day in your recovery. What behaviors seemed to keep you* ***feeling crummy****? Lying? So, if you want to have a 3 star day tomorrow, how long will you have to lie in order to do that?"* In their own special ways, they'll get the same point.

The disease behaviors that they insist on keeping are their character defects.

Have them circle one character defect.

To end the group, have each client identify one disease behavior they notice **already beginning to end.** Are they willing to practice letting go of it completely for 24 hours?

Then identify one recovery behavior that was **easy for them to do.** Would they like to practice this consistently for 24 hours?

Remind the group that we work with one step at a time, one behavior at a time, and one day at a time. How do we eat an elephant? One bite at a time!

(Getting out of . . . .)

THE EXPECTATION TRAP

Group warm-up introduction:

Chemically dependent people hate reality. "Drugs are for people who can't stand reality." Remember that?

While **we end up using** alcohol because we have to, **we start off using** it to alter our reality. We use to feel better, to escape our pain or discomfort, or to take a break from "life", whatever that is. When we quit using, we are still trapped in that cycle: *Our reality does not match our expectations.* This is evident in the belief that in order "to be happy," we would like to be someplace else emotionally, physically, financially, and so forth. How many of us still say, "I wish I were" . . . ."if only" . . . ."if I could just" . . . "winning the lottery" . . .

Pass out the story in Handout #31: I Wish, I Wish, I Wish to the group. Have one member read it .

All of these "wishes" and "desires" are a good way to get loaded. It follows this simple formula:

(Please place the diagram on the blackboard in numerical order. Draw out the lines.)

1. My "wishes" are up here.______________________________________

} **3. This space in between here is the difference between our expectations and reality. It is filled with feelings that we can get drunk over — frustration, despair, anxiety, shame, loneliness, "I hate myself", etc.**

2. My reality is down here.______________________________________

Now that we are clean and sober, we still have this split between *what we wish* and *our reality.* We still have those dangling feelings **shown above in #3** floating around in our emotional space.

To alleviate those uncomfortable feelings, we have two options:

1. We can get loaded again which may numb out those feelings in space #3.

2. We can lower Line #1 down to Line #2, **close the gap in #3,** to reduce those negative and harmful feelings.

Materials Needed: Chalkboard, Handout - "I Wish, I Wish, I Wish"

The group exercise:

Ask for a volunteer: Client #1

Step #1: Have Client #1 write 8-10 of their **wishes** on the board horizontally along the "I Wish" line.

Step #2: Well below the list, have them list their corresponding **realities**.

Step #3: Ask the client to identify their **feelings** in Space #3.

STEP #1	I WISH:	I were pretty	I was rich	I had a girlflfriend	I was not an alcoholic

feeling ________ ex. feeling shame ← STEP #3 - *Have the client identify the feelings they have in the disparity between what they wish & reality*

STEP #2	MY REALITY:	I look OK	I have $300	I'm single	I am alcoholic

To lessen the uncomfortable feelings in Space #3, we need to lower Space #1.

The only way to do this is to accept reality.

Remind them that all of the wishes in Space#1 are outside things. Recovery is an inside job — ***It's about working with the feeling's Space in #3, not getting Space #1 to be happy!***

In Space #1, **the wishes never end** — there is never enough money, or pretty enough, or the perfect girlfriend. *This is also part of our insanity in Step Two.*

Ask Client #1 to go back through their list again, **this time re-examining their reality.** What is okay about having $300.00, being single, and so forth? How are these things good and perfect for them at this time?

What is the hidden gift in each aspect of their reality? What spiritual lessons are to be found in each of these gifts? How does accepting reality alter the amount of painful feelings in space #3?

Repeat with each group member.

Follow-up — process some of these ideas:

- Having done this exercise, what's happened to your feelings in that empty space?
- How does **acceptance** help you?
- Can you practice this just for today?
- How can this be a tool for society?

HANDOUT #31

I WISH, I WISH, I WISH

One day God miraculously appeared to Michael and said, "My child, I love you deeply and completely. However, I spend so much time listening to you pray for this and for that, that I do not have time for my other responsibilities. To resolve this problem, I will grant you three wishes. Anything you wish will come true, but you will be given only three wishes to last this lifetime."

Naturally, Michael carefully considered wishes about immense wealth, power, perfect health, and so forth. The truth was that Michael was an honest and caring man. So, he finally decided that his true happiness lay close to his heart and that perfect love was his first wish. Unable to divorce in this country, he wished that his nagging wife would die peacefully in her sleep and be carried off by a sweet angel who would love her in heaven. He would then be free to make his second wish for that perfect love to appear.

After his wife died, his children were inconsolable. They wept for days, especially the baby who needed her mother and his son who adored her. He was able to see what he could not see before. His wife had been precious in her own way. He came to realize that while he had hated her nagging and all of her faults, he missed her too. So, he wished for her to return from heaven.

For months and months, Michael was unable to decide what to wish for last. He asked his friends, the village priest, and his parents for advice. He consulted oracles and gypsy fortune tellers and was still distraught. He needed money to provide for his family, he longed for a perfect and healthy body, and he wished his children to be happy all of their lives.

Finally, in great despair, he came across an old man sitting quietly in the sun. When asked why he looked so miserable, he sat and told his story to the ancient one. "Ah," smiled the old man gently, "The only way out of your dilemma is to wish for acceptance. That you will be content and recognize all of the things in your life as a gift, no matter what."

PEER GROUP - TOUGH LOVE

This is a tough group to do right. Done badly, this group can emotionally devastate and wound your patients by thoughtlessly shaming and degrading them. Done carefully and with sensitivity, this group can create immense self-esteem, reward difficult and painful work, and assist the client in making choices about how to get "unstuck" in their denial. *Always use a co-therapist sitting across from you to provide safety for the group.*

"Peer feedback" is always heard more deeply than "counselor feedback". When the client hears something from a friend in treatment, it has a much more profound impact on them than feedback from the therapist.

The goals of this group are many. **The primary goal** is to allow your client to hear an honest assessment from their group about where they are in treatment. They will get their treatment status reflected to them in these two areas:

1. **The ways I see you growing are ______________________.**
2. **The ways I see you holding back are __________________.**

A second goal is for the group participants. Individuals within the group are given an opportunity to develop their skills in being assertive — saying what they mean without being judgmental or passive.

The task for the therapist is to be able to guide the group in such a manner that the client can hear where they are lacking in recovery without experiencing shame. This is also a good method to take the temperature of the group by observing their interactions and manner of confrontation, (i.e., who is the group's hero, scapegoat, etc., and to see who needs to grow assertively).

The group format is very simple.

Start the group with the introduction that the group is called **Tough Love** for two reasons:

1. It is tough to **hear** honest feedback **from** people you care about.
2. It is tough **giving** honest feedback **to** somebody you care about.

Instruct the group on "feedback guidelines." The group members are to provide feedback to each other in two areas:

The way I see you growing is________________

The way I see you holding back is_____________

Note:

For both areas of feedback, they are only allowed to point out clients' ***behaviors and they must give an example.*** Feedback without an example is vague and meaningless. Identifying **only** examples of **behaviors** keeps judgment and second guessing out of the group dynamic and reduces personal shame.

Keep the feedback to under 90 seconds per person.

No advice may be given at any time by anybody, *including the therapists.* **(No "shoulds.")** Advice giving places the client in a double-bind. In explaining this rule, ask the group to give examples of what they have experienced when given advice. They'll get the point.

Inform the group that your role and the counselor's role includes giving feedback, but *is mainly to provide emotional safety for the group.* To provide emotional safety means interrupting and redirecting judgmental statements (shaming messages), and interrupting advice-giving by having the group reframe their feedback to the client.

You might also ask for more specific examples.

Example of "Tough Love Feedback".

"Mary, ***the ways I see you growing are many.*** *The denial you had about how much and how long you used seems to be gone.* ***For example,*** *"I heard you talking honestly about how much you drank in group yesterday and on your Step One. You were less defensive. Today, I saw you spending more time with your peers and isolating less.* ***The way I see you holding back is*** *that you still have not shared in AA".*

Note:

- **Try to give two or more examples of growth.**
- Give **only one** example of holding back. It can be too overwhelming to give more than one example of denial and will shame the client.
- Keep the feedback simple. Do not allow group members to use platitudes like — "I know you are strong and you can handle it". It is cheap and ingratiating. Stick to straight feedback.
- Ask the group if they have questions.
- Show them examples of feedback and proper body position. (See below.)

To start the group, ask who would like to **receive** feedback first, Client A.

Ask Client A to place both feet on the ground, hands on either leg, take a deep breath, and give eye contact at all times to the people giving feedback. **This is an open position which keeps clients open to feedback. Crossed arms allows them to defend against honesty.**

The person to their left, Client B, gives Client A feedback. Client B signals that they are finished, when they say "That 's it".

Then Client C gives Client A feedback, etc., until the circle is complete.

Only at this point may Client A respond, (after everybody has given them feedback).

> Client A responds in a **general way** about what they heard in the two areas of feedback, i.e., *"I heard people say that the way I am growing is that I am isolating less and have moved through a lot of my denial. The way that I am holding back is by not speaking in AA"*.

They may not refute or attack the feedback or those giving it, i.e., *"Robert, you were wrong when you said that I didn't talk at AA, and Amy, what do you know about my family"*, etc.

Only a **general response** to what they hear the **group** say is permitted.

Following Client A's summary of their feedback, ask him:

What his commitment is that week to working on "how he is holding back."?

How will the group see that he is actually working on it? (It needs to be measurable.)

Example:

> "I heard people say I minimized the effect my drinking had on my kids. I will talk about it in group **tomorrow** and bring it up in the family meeting on Wednesday".

Always honor their commitment. Do not try to change it or add to it. They are telling you about the level of the coping tools they have to change.

Then, Client B receives feedback.

Complete the circle.

When the group is finished, clients may feel isolated and vulnerable. To close the group, do something warm to bring the group together.

Compliment them all on having stayed in the group and for being honest; that this was hard.

Close with a serenity prayer or group hug. This brings the isolate back into the group.

Hints:

1. If somebody has only one week in treatment, they will not know how to give feedback yet, and they will not know their peers well. They only receive *fairly superficial* feedback and do not give feedback.

2. Do not allow "therapy" in the Tough Love Group. It will sabotage the group by breaking the rules and by giving extra attention to the personality disorders who tend to distort groups. Issues always come up as a result of this group so......

3. Do this group in the morning. Follow-up with group therapy to process feelings or issues that surfaced for them. Always allow for a follow-up group.

4. Plan a hidden agenda with your co-therapist before group. This group can be very powerful for these two reasons: First,

   If you want to make a point, different people repeating the exact same feedback is very powerful. If ten people tell me that I have denial about abusing my wife, **and that's all they say,** then chances are that I will hear it.

   Secondly, it is an excellent tool for working with personality disorders. Paradox them in a positive way. If you have a narcissist who constantly interrupts others and focuses the group on themselves, feedback could go something like this — "*When you first came here, you used to interrupt everybody and turn the attention to yourself. It was very difficult to let Mary get the time she needed.* ***The way I see you growing is*** *that you did not interrupt her. You gave her the space she needed in group yesterday. I see you growing with more respect and insight for others.* ***The way I see you holding back is*** *by not talking more about what is going on for you when you interrupt others. I would like to hear about that*".

   Do the same things with sociopathic clients. Give them positive feedback for being less threatening, manipulative, etc. Give a specific example and ask for more disclosure which will have them look at their underlying issues to become part of the group emotionally.

5. Try to keep feedback positive and install healthy ego strengths.
This avoids destroying any trust they have been able to build. The tougher they look, the more fragile they are. Do some nurturing.

For example: *"When you were admitted you were defensive and lied about everything. I'm really amazed and impressed by how you've been able to let down that mask. You were really sensitive to Mary in group yesterday when you . . . .".*

- This group is best done weekly.
- Let the older group members explain how the group works to the newcomers.
- Ask if someone else would like to fill in some details or explanations when they are finished explaining.
- See if the group has questions.
- Define your role again.

SOCIAL ATOMS

Social atoms helps clients use physical action, rather than narrative, to explore the network of significant others in their lives.

Individual Goal: Understanding where we stand with the significant people in our lives is the first step to accepting the role alcoholism and addiction plays in distancing us from others. Are people moving toward us or away from us? What are the messages the important people in our lives have for us? What feelings are stirred by examining and recreating our relationships?

Group Goal: Group cohesion is developed through individual self-disclosure, peer support, and the consideration of the depth of the needs and feelings of others.

Materials needed: A large group room, drawing materials, Blackboard.

Action:

1. The counselor uses the blackboard to diagram the social network of a fictional client.

2. In the center of the atom diagram is a little circle (or other geometric figure) to represent the client.

3. Surrounding this center little circle are 3 to 10 significant others (also represented by geometric figures).

4. These significant others can include relatives, friends, pets, addictive substances, and people who are no longer living but continue to play a role in the client's life. If clients have many significant others, it is an interesting exercise to have them choose the most important ones.

5. Clients judge the distance between themselves and their significant others **by how close they feel to that person.** Lines can be drawn to each of the significant others to indicate whether the feelings are positive, negative, or neutral.

6. After the example atom has been explained, clients are invited to draw their own.

7. When everyone is finished, ask for sharing from the group.

Sample of a Social Atom:

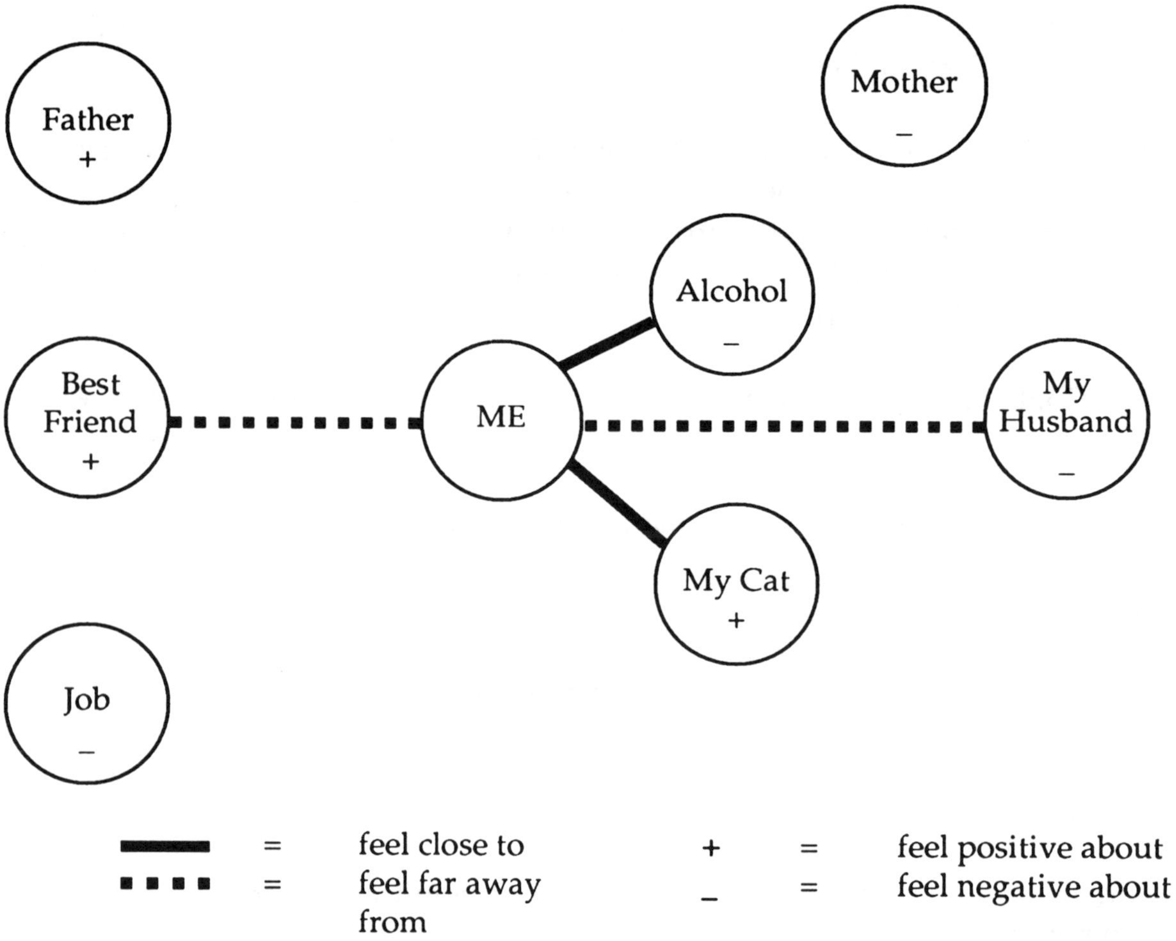

Suggestion:

Depending on the functioning level of the group, this exercise can be expanded by **putting the atom into action:**

1. Invite a high functioning client, Tom, to select another group member to represent him in the center of the atom. It must never be assumed that the peer will be willing to take on this role. He must be asked.

2. If the group member agrees, ask him to represent Tom.

3. Tom then takes the role of a sculptor. Tom as the sculptor then invites other group members, one at a time, to represent the significant others in his life.

4. Tom can give even more clarity to the atom by physically sculpting the significant others into statues.

5. After all the significant others are molded into a body position and at a distance which satisfies Tom, he returns to the center of the atom sculpture.

6. From the perspective of the center position, Tom may want to make further changes to more exactly recreate the picture of his life.

7. Instruct Tom to sculpt the atom by instinct rather than intellect. Allow him to create an atom which feels true.

An additional element can now be added:

1. Ask Tom to leave the center of the atom and replace himself with the original group member.

2. Instruct Tom to go to each statue and give that significant other a line of dialogue that they may typically say. *"What is the most important message this person gives you?"* So if Tom has somebody representing his mother, ask Tom to switch roles with that person who is acting as his mother. Now Tom is "Mother."

3. Ask "Mother" to make one statement about Tom. For example: *"Tom, you're always late," or "Tom, you're my favorite son."*

4. Have Tom switch back with the first person who was "Mother."

5. Tom now switches roles with another person in his sculpture.

6. After all the messages are given out, the client again returns to the center position and listens to the messages one at a time, furthest away and toward the center.

7. These messages may also be "flooded" by instructing the significant others to all speak their messages at once.

Ample time for sharing and group process should be given. It is not necessary that all the clients complete every stage of this expanded exercise.

- **What feelings did peer group members experience watching the work?**

- **What was it like playing a significant other?** It can sometimes be painful to play a more negative role.

- **What feelings did you experience?**

- **Will continued sobriety change the structure, shape and messages of the atom?**

HANDOUT #32

DRAW YOUR SOCIAL ATOM:

THREE CHAIR EXERCISE

A sober qualification is based on an alcoholics personal story of:

- What it was like.
- What happened.
- What it is like now.

In the "Three-Chair Exercise" the concept of sobriety as a journey is introduced.

Individual Goal: Why am I afraid to let you know who I really am? To place our dreams before the crowd is to risk. The greatest risk of all, however, is the opportunity not taken. Through self-disclosure, clients learn trust and develop a sense of sobriety as a journey.

Group goal: Increased intimacy and trust among peers.

Materials needed: Three chairs in the front of the room facing the group.

Action: The "Three-Chair Exercise" explores:

- What life used to be like.
- What life is like now.
- What the future may hold.

The chairs individually represent a moment from the past, a moment in the present, and a moment in the future.

Warm-Up: A guided imagery to explore the past, present, and future. Ask clients to relax, close their eyes, and breathe deeply.

Read Slowly And Calmly*. Pause between sentences. Allow five minutes for this reading:*

There is no right or wrong way to follow this exploratory exercise. Each of us is different, with a different past, a different present reality, and a different future. All of us, however, have the possibility of a sober future. And, we are sober now. Right in this very moment. Sober.

Now relaxing deeply and following my voice, I am going to ask you some questions. These will be questions to think about deep inside.

Allow yourself to shift your body position so that you are comfortable. Breathe deeply. Now, think about a specific moment from your past. Just one moment.

How old are you? Picture the place where you are living. Take your time so that you can really see it. In this one moment from your past, who are the people in your life?

Now, picture yourself. What is important to you now? Is drinking or doing other drugs a part of your picture? In this one moment from your past what do you want for your life?

Allow for a few moments of quiet before moving on.

Now, breathe deeply and allow yourself to move into the present moment. This specific moment in time. Right now. Right here.

Who are the people in your life right now? Now picture yourself. What is important to you in this moment in time? Is drinking or doing other drugs a part of the picture? In this moment, this very moment, what do you want for your life?

Pause for a few minutes.

Now, when you are ready, breathe deeply and move into a place in your future. One specific moment that has yet to be. Do so at your own pace.

What is your life like right now? Who is in your life? Picture yourself in this moment in the future. What is important to you? What is your relationship to alcohol and other drugs in this moment. What are your hopes right now?

Pause for a few minutes.

Now, when you are ready, prepare yourself to open your eyes and rejoin the group. Feel your feet on the floor allow yourself to stretch and open your eyes. Now you are back in the room.

Follow-Up:
The counselor invites each client to individually share from the chairs in the front of the room representing the past, the present, and a moment from the future. *No processing, just a statement.*

After this exercise, ample time for group process is important. Clients can be encouraged to share from a feeling level about both their own experience with the exercise and about the experience of witnessing the work of their peers.

Feedback should be directed to what the audience saw, heard, and felt the client in the front of the room saying, keeping advice out.

HONESTY

"Those who do not recover are constitutionally incapable of being honest with themselves." (Chapter 5, "How It Works", Alcoholic Anonymous.) This presentation explores the value of "getting real" about ourselves and our process.

Individual Goal: Clients will disclose information about themselves and recognize the importance of rigorous honesty in their recovery.

Group Goal: To admit to not telling the truth, to lying, can often prove to be a shame-provoking experience. This group uses play as an emotional paradox. At the end of this group, clients may proclaim, *"This group is a bunch of terrific liars. We are some of the best liars in the world!"* Acknowledging what is **not** true can serve as a beginning to what is. At the very least, it opens group members to listening for the truth.

The Presentation:

Warm-up discussion: Honesty is essential for a recovery program. Honesty, Openness, Willingness. The "Big Book" of Alcoholics Anonymous is riddled with references to rigorous honesty. *"Rarely have we seen a person fail who has thoroughly followed our path. Those who do not recover are usually men and women who are constitutionally incapable of being honest with themselves. They are not at fault. They seem to have been born that way."*

Group warmup: What are some possible pay-offs to being honest, telling the truth?

Sobriety
Higher self-esteem
Less tension
Self-respect

Each pay-off needs a specific example from a client's personal experience in being honest.

Warm-Up Game: Two Truths And A Lie

This game is a fun way to help clients begin to differentiate between truth and falsehood.

The group forms a circle.

Instruct the group to think about three statements — two being true and one being totally dishonest. The more outrageous the better.

The goal of the game is to see if you can fool the group.

After a client has disclosed his/her three statements the group votes, one at a time, for the false statement.

The counselor can model the action of the game by going first in a sample round.

Example: One of these statements is untrue. Which one is it?

A. *"I once melted rum raisin ice cream on a Sunday night when the bars were closed and I had no money, just to get a drink."*

B. *"I once appeared on a television game show, terribly hung over, and lost in front of millions of people."*

C. *"I once nearly drowned on a Colorado River rafting trip trying to save the pot in by backpack when it fell overboard."*

If the counselor models statements concerning pre-recovery issues, the clients will be more inclined to identify information regarding their own using histories. This game is not about 'war stories', **it is about the ease of not telling the truth**. The counselor need not be a recovering alcoholic addict. The truths and lies need to address behavior, however.

After everyone has had a turn, hold a discussion:

- Who in the group fooled the most people?
- What techniques do you use to keep people from determining the truth?
- How was your eye contact? Body Language?
- Were the techniques you used in the game the same as the ones you use in "real life"?

By the way, if you chose C, your powers of determining the truth are extraordinary. I would be a better sober bank robber than a drunk one. In sobriety, choices are increased.

Here is another game, designed to prompt more discussion about honesty and to build on the energy of **"Two Truths And A Lie"**

To Tell The Truth

This game is similar to the old television game show.
Set three chairs in front of the room facing the group.
Divide the group into groups of three.

Instruct the first team to come up with a story. The story should be true for one person and a lie for the two other people. The team goal is to fool the rest of the group.

The first team leaves the room and has 5 minutes to develop their story.

When they return, they take chairs in the front of the room and, one at a time, briefly tell the story:

Example:

- *"My name is Bob, and what I am going to tell you is true. It happened to me."*
- *"My name is Joan, and this really, truly happened . . ."*
- *"My name is Terry, and no matter what the others tell you, I am the one telling the truth. Believe me when I tell you . . ."*

The group has up to six questions to ask the individuals on the panel in order to help them identify the truth teller.

The group then votes on the person telling the truth.

"Would the real truth teller please stand up?"

Prolonging the suspense, the truth teller stands and the counselor leads the applause. Paradoxical affirmations of the group members' lying abilities can keep the game flowing and fast paced.

Use the 5 minute break times to hold free form discussions about characteristics of honesty.

- We have a choice to be honest.
- It is important to be honest about our motives.
- Small lies are lies, too.
- It can be risky to honestly confront others on their behavior.
- Honesty can be used as a mask to hide hostility or nastiness, etc.

The break times can also be used to relay information about honesty and dishonesty. Use the blackboard to record this information:

1. **Lying can be direct. Lying by commission.**

   For example: *"I am a professional basketball player. Oh, and I also hold the world record for the 100 yard dash. I speak fluent Chinese."*

2. **Lying can be indirect. Lying by omission**. These are the things we do not say in order to mislead others. It is the information we conveniently leave out.

   For example: *"Does anyone know who ate the last piece of pie?"* If you ate the pie and you do not say anything, you are lying by omission.

3. **Collusion** is when more than one person shares a lie. It is a secret agreement. Sometimes families suffering from alcoholism collude around the lie, *"Everything is really okay in our family."*

After the last team has presented, review the information on the board so that everyone, especially those people who were out of the room, has a clear understanding.

Being dishonest can be a set-up for using.

Assignment for the next group. *"What untruth, no matter how small, have you told today"?* This includes lies of commission, lies of omission, and colluding.

Close the group with a confidentiality circle.

"What you heard here, when you leave here, let it stay here."

LIFELINE

The lifeline shows your clients how the various parts of their story fit together. It helps them to concretize their work in treatment by weaving together sections of their Step One and other groups.

This group is usually done toward the end of treatment when the client has much more insight into the dynamics of their addiction. Their lifeline allows the client to see the whole picture of their story, to practice telling their story, and to experience positive reinforcement for their insight and honesty.

Materials Needed: Very large sheet of paper, colored markers, Handout # 33

Review the Lifeline Handout with the group.

Have clients create their individual Lifelines.

Follow-up Group: The client tapes their lifeline to a wall. Remind them that they are "telling their story" so their lifeline review needs to remain under 20 minutes.

In the remaining time, allow the group to give feedback and ask questions:

- How thorough did they find the presentation?
- Did they see any denial?
- What stage of recovery do they think he/she's in?

Variations: Depending upon the focus of your treatment center, you may have the client begin their lifeline at birth, adding more pertinent data about their history of abuse, development of codependency, eating disorders, etc. For the dually diagnosed client, they may add the progression of their mental illness.

HANDOUT #33

LIFELINE

This is your lifeline. It gives you the opportunity to gather the different aspects of your addiction into one story. You will be examining your story related to how you were **feeling** during your years of addiction and the **events** going on.

On a large sheet of paper, set up a graph. The vertical line is your **feeling meter**. The horizontal line going across from left to right is the **time line, your age.**

The following are suggestions only: You may add in your own feeling words but keep feeling "normal" in the middle.

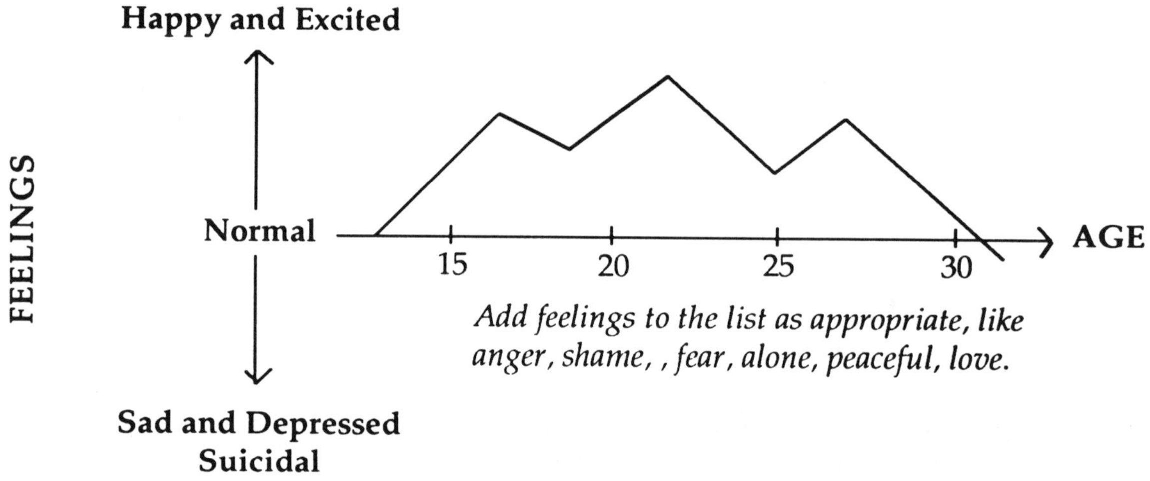

Begin your time line with when you started drinking/using. Make sure you have at least 8 marks along your time line.

These marks will indicate the number of years that you used until you came into this treatment program. So, if you drank for 16 years, and you need 8 marks on the graph, each mark will indicate 2 years of your life. You can add in more years on the graph or change it around as you need.

For example: If you started drinking when you were 16 and things stayed pretty much the same until you were 20, the next marker and explanation will be 4 years later, at age 20. There needs to be a minimum of 8 to 10 markers, (or ages).

1. Start with your drinking and using line. Show your history of drinking and using and how you felt during those years.

2. Using a different colored pencil, draw in your job line and how you felt during those ages. Feel free to change the feelings on the graph and add your own. These are only suggestions.

3. Continue with different colored pencils, mapping out these areas or events in your life:

   - Drinking/Using History
   - Job History
   - Finances
   - When were your children born?
   - Social Life
   - Health
   - Legal Issues
   - Relationships — All marriages, divorces, relationships, etc.

Add events that were important to you.

For most of us, the first years of our drinking and using were good and our life seemed to be on an upswing. Be able to indicate this and to show how things in your life started changing.

Show the how and why of the changes.

FOLLOWING DIRECTIONS: THE ROAD MAP TO RECOVERY

Objectives:

1. To help clients identify the value of following directions.

2. To reinforce recovery directions and rationale.

3. To challenge the client to make a specific commitment to one of the directions he is not following.

Materials needed: Blackboard, Handout # 34 —"Can You Follow Directions?", pencils.

Pass out the Handout— "Can You Follow Directions?" to all members. Tell the group to follow the directions as they are written.

Allow ten minutes for completion of the assignment. **Give no further directions.**

Reconvene the group. If they are laughing, tell them you have decided not to ask any of them to assemble your new bicycle! Go around the group so each member can describe their experience, and have them include which directions they did not follow.

Take a few minutes to have volunteers describe a time when not following directions backfired.

What are some of the thoughts that come up when members are given directions? **Examples:**

- "I don't need directions, I can figure it out myself."
- "Don't insult my intelligence."
- "I know what works for me."
- "I don't like to be told what to do or how to do it."
- "My way or no way."
- "You take the high road and I'll take the low road."
- "When all else fails maybe I'll try directions."
- "I don't do anything I don't agree with."
- "Oh yeah? Do it yourself!"

Doesn't the hair on your neck just raise up a little when someone else suggests what you should do? How can all of this affect our recovery? Here's the news about suggestions and recovery. The good news is: **It is absolutely rare that anyone who follows the recovery directions will get drunk or use.** The bad news is: **Alcoholics and addicts are terrible at following directions!**

Have you noticed that AA has suggestions for staying sober?
Let's make a list on the blackboard and discuss them. The list will be called Directions: The Road Map to Recovery.

As we go along, notice the ones you are following, those you are working on, and *any that just don't apply to you at all.*

What is the first and primary suggestion in AA?

1. **Don't drink and go to meetings** (90 meetings in 90 days).

***Note: It is important that this be the first on the list. Additions can be added by the group but this must be #1.**

Ask members to share specific ways that going to meetings is helping them to stay sober.

> **The facts:** People who attend meetings regularly tend to stay sober. Attending 90 meetings in 90 days takes commitment to sobriety, and is "doable" if we decide to do it. Meetings, in most areas, are available to fit any daily schedule. In early recovery, AA members who do not attend meetings usually relapse.
>
> The suggestion does not mean that we have to like meetings. We just go anyway, whether we like them or not. Many alcoholics have described hating meetings, and are sober and alive to tell about it.
>
> If you are convinced that AA is not for you but you really want to stay sober, then you have the right intention and motivation. You may be in denial about how to achieve it. If you really are serious about recovery then try this: Write down your argument about not needing AA and present to the group. If none of these denial experts find a hint of denial, go for it. Otherwise, strongly consider changing your mind. It could save your life.

2. **Get a sponsor and have regular contact.**

3. **Work the steps with a sponsor.**

Note: Combining #'s 2 and 3 impresses on clients that the Steps must be worked with a sponsor. If the group has not had a sponsorship lecture, they will have lots of questions and concerns about finding a sponsor. For now you can just include a few facts.

The facts: The 12 Steps of AA were written and designed as a way of sober living with a support system built in. The steps begin with the pronoun, "We". The recovering alcoholic's strength lies in her connection to other alcoholics. We do not stay sober alone. We stay sober together!

A sponsor is an AA member who has experience in sobriety and has worked the steps with her sponsor. Does everyone in AA meet these criteria? Unfortunately not. Since the only requirement for AA membership is a desire to stop drinking, we have to search some for a person who follows these very suggestions. "Stick with the winners." Choosing a sponsor is an important decision, and we need help and information to make a wise choice. AA has a pamphlet on sponsorship which is helpful and is available in most Central Service Offices. Ask for help in choosing a sponsor!

4. **Join a home group.** Making sober friends is no small task. Join a regular group and commit to attending that meeting weekly along with taking some responsibility, like volunteering for a particular task within the group. This can really help us in getting to know and socialize with other members.

5. **Prayer and meditation:** Ask the members if they have found a spiritual practice that is working for them. How does it help you in your sobriety?

The facts: AA is not a religion. There are no rules on spirituality. Your personal sense and development of spirituality will grow with you in recovery.

Some of us choose to return to religious practices while others turn to the powers of nature. However you come to practice prayer, just remember to keep it very simple by asking something bigger than yourself to keep you sober for "today" and then thank "it" at the end of that sober day. You do not have to understand or know what "it" is. The only sure thing that most of us do know and understand is that we could not stop using on our own.

To practice meditation in its simplest form is to be quiet and allow the mind a break from our busy and constant thinking. You will find the prayer and meditation practices that suit you. A sponsor can be a helpful resource.

6. **AA service:** What ways can you give in AA?

The facts: There are a number of ways to be of service in AA such as: Making coffee, setting up meeting rooms, reaching out your hand and welcoming newcomers, chairing at a meeting, and answering phones at the area Central Office. The saying in AA is *"You can't keep it unless you give it away."*

7. **Read The Big Book.** When you read *The Big Book and The Twelve and Twelve*, take what fits and leave the rest. Amazingly for many of us, as we read it again, more and more seems to fit.

Continue the list to include suggestions from the group like: "Let Go And Let God," asking for help, and changing playmates, play things and play pens.

Have the group briefly describe how these tools work for them.

End the group by having each member make a specific commitment addressing one suggestion they have not followed as yet. **Example:** *"I will have a sponsor by Monday." "I will read my meditation book every morning this week." "I will spend 15 minutes a day reading The Big Book."*

HANDOUT #34

CAN YOU FOLLOW DIRECTIONS?

1. Read everything carefully before doing anything.
2. Put your name in the upper right hand corner of this paper.
3. Draw five small squares in the upper left hand corner.
4. Put an "X" in each square.
5. Put a circle around each square.
6. Sign you name under the title of the paper.
7. After the title, write "yes, yes, yes."
8. Put a circle completely around sentence number 7.
9. Put an "X" in the lower left corner of this page.
10. Draw a triangle around the "X" you just put down.
11. On the back of this paper, multiply 703 by 66
12. Draw a rectangle around the corner in sentence 4
13. When you get this far hold up your right arm.
14. If you have followed directions carefully to this point, stand up.
15. On the reverse side of this paper add 8950 and 9805.
16. Put a circle around your answer and put a square around the circle.
17. On the right side of your paper write the numbers 10 to 1 backwards.
18. Punch three small holes in the top of this paper with your pencil point.
19. Underline all even numbers on the left side of this paper.
20. Wave both arms in the air.
21. Now that you have finished reading everything carefully, do only sentence 1 and 2 and then sit quietly until the others have finished.

AA QUESTIONS, QUESTIONS, QUESTIONS

This is a simple group that answers often asked questions about Twelve Step Recovery. The facilitator of the group should be a staff member who is engaged in Twelve Step Recovery themselves and can clarify information or answer questions which arise in the group.

Ask the group to sit in a circle.

On Handout #35 you will find a list of questions which can be copied, cut and attached to 3x5 index cards. The index cards are distributed to group members, with instructions to keep them face down.

Instructions: On the cards you will find questions about recovery. A volunteer will begin by turning over a card and reading the question. He will choose a peer in the group to respond. If the respondent is not sure of an answer, **he must make a guess.** *"I don't know"* is not allowed as a response. Other group members may then contribute information they feel is relevant to the question. The facilitator then will clarify information as needed, and move on to the next question.

Note: The facilitator's role should be minimal and objective.

For example: *"Now that is a very interesting concept. Here is the suggestion in recovery ____________________ and here is the idea behind it __________________."*

Allow clients to get a little silly and have some fun!

HANDOUT #35

AA QUESTIONS

What do you do if you run into someone you know at a meeting?

How do you find a sponsor and what do you look for in a sponsor?

If you are doing 90/90 and you miss a meeting, what do you do?

If your partner and you are both in recovery, do you go to the same meetings?

What does "Trying's Lying" mean?

What is 13th Stepping?

When do you start your 4th Step?

What is "Two Stepping"?

What does "Live and Let Live" mean?

You are a heroin addict. Can you go to AA?

Can you go to a meeting drunk?

Where is the best place to sit in a meeting?

Do you speak more than once in an AA meeting?

Explain what "Principles before Personalities" means.

What does anonymity mean to you?

What does "Keep It Simple" mean?

Where does the money go in AA?

Why is the "Newcomer" the most important person in the room?

What does "Thinking through the Drink" mean?

How often can you go to the bar now that you are sober?

What is "Keeping it Green"?

If you were to relapse, "Who ya gonna call?"

Can you speak at a Step 6 meeting if you have not done the sixth step?

How do you "fire" a sponsor?

What is isolating?

How often do you call a sponsor?

What is a drunkalog?

What is page 449 in the Big Book?

What is "being on the pity pot?"

What is a Twelfth Step call?

What is the best way to convince a using friend to go to a meeting?

What does "attraction rather than promotion" mean to you?

What is "Stinkin Thinkin?"

What is resentment? And what can you do about it?

What is a home group? Why do we need one?

What kind of service can newcomers do?

What do you do if you can't reach your sponsor?

Who is the sickest person at any meeting?

When do you start going to other types of 12 Step meetings, like Al-Anon?

Does a therapy session count as a meeting?

What do they talk about in Men's and Women's groups?

If you break your leg, how do you get to a meeting?

What are the AA Promises?

What are the only requirements for AA?

Why do they say "The most expensive cigarettes are sold in liquor stores," even if they are giving them away for free?

What is a good day for an alcoholic?

Why do we say there are no "slips" in AA?

What does "There are no accidents" mean?

Why do they say "You can always pee in a gas station, not in a bar"?

What is the short form of the Serenity Prayer?

What is an AA miracle?

Why do they say "Make sobriety your top priority"?

Why do they say "You didn't get sick overnight"?

Why do they say "The only difference between a recovered and recovering alcoholic is that a recovering alcoholic is still breathing?"

Who needs to know you are an alco-holic?

When are the two times to go to a meeting?

Why would somebody tell you to "take the cotton out of your ears and stick it in your mouth"?

What are Beginner's Meetings?

SPEAKING IN AA

Objective: To allow clients to explore the issues, fears, and concerns they have about raising their hands and sharing in AA.

Taking responsibility for becoming a part of AA is no small task for alcoholics. For most of us, isolation is the common rule. Engaging with other alcoholics is a milestone in early recovery, and for most of us it takes guts and humility.

Recovering alcoholics are very aware of the difficulty newcomers have in starting their programs. In most meetings as part of the opening process, newcomers are invited to introduce themselves. The suggestion is to take advantage of this opportunity for the first 30 days of sobriety. We get some practice at raising our hands and other members come to know us by name.

1. Ask the group what comes up for them when they raise their hand and speak in AA.

> **Examples:** *"I get too nervous." "I don't know what to say." "My voice shakes." "I'm afraid I'll say the wrong thing." "I'm too new to sobriety, I have nothing important to say." "I'm ashamed to be in an AA meeting."*

As newcomers to AA, we can feel a little lost. The language sometimes sounds foreign. Words like *"drunkalog", "bottom", "sign-post", and "Higher Power"* can leave us feeling left in the dark. Although there are no directions given about how an AA meeting works, after we've attended a few meetings we get the idea that there are some unspoken rules that exist.

There are usually three types of meetings available and your area AA Schedules will indicate the type of meeting:

- **Speaker meeting**
- **Discussion meeting**
- **Step meeting**

In Speaker's meetings, a person has already been designated to share. The directions on being the speaker are outlined in *"How It Works"* in Chapter 5 of The Big Book. This is sometimes called a "Drunkalog." We share what it was like (our using/drinking story), what happened (how we got sober), and what it is like today (our sobriety now).

Most groups through group conscience will have guidelines about how much sober or clean time a member needs to have before they are a meeting speaker. Often the guideline is 90 days. The reason for this is that if I'm a newcomer then I am probably not experienced about the *"getting sober"* phase. So, there is the first guideline: **If I am not the speaker then I don't have to give a drunkalog in the meeting.** Does every newcomer know this? No, so if I start giving my using history are you going to judge me? Hopefully not, and I will catch on with a little time. Is it okay if I have done that already? Absolutely.

The Discussion and Step meetings usually have an opening speaker and then the meetings are open to sharing from any member.

Here are a few guidelines for sharing that you may find useful.

1. Speak in the "I." Since AA has no opinions, in my sharing I own **my** experience and opinions. I don't state "facts." Someone else's experience and opinion may be different from mine.

2. We avoid giving feedback in AA. We do not comment about what you say in a way which assumes judgment, or which gives advice. AA is not the same as group therapy, nor is it the place to agree or disagree with someone else. Feedback is important in my recovery, and my sponsor and sober friends can play a helpful role in that area.

   Limit your sharing to a few minutes. We listen, thank the person for sharing and share our own experience.

So, now what can you share at meetings?

3. Generate a list of topics from the group. Allow for brief discussion on each example.

   Use this time to help the group explore their anxiety or resistance. When they express concerns, suggest that their concerns are all appropriate topics in AA.

HANDOUT #36

SPEAKING IN AA

TOPICS I CAN TALK ABOUT AT AN AA MEETING :

Difficulty I have in raising my hand to speak.

Cravings, urges to drink.

Using dreams.

Resistance to coming to meetings.

Difficulty asking someone to be my sponsor.

Problems calling my sponsor.

Feelings.

Boredom.

Dealing with using friends or relatives.

Sober experiences (things I have done for the first time sober).

Isolating behavior.

Making sober friends.

Breaking through denial.

Consequences of my using.

The steps.

Relapse.

Old behaviors.

New behaviors.

Changes in sobriety.

My relationship with my Higher Power.

THINGS THAT BUG ME ABOUT AA MEETINGS

Introduction:

For alcoholics and addicts, engaging in a Twelve Step Recovery Program affords the greatest opportunity for continued sobriety. This is not so easy. Resistance to AA is significant early in recovery. At this stage there is discomfort about being with a group of strangers and a tendency to compare rather than identify with others in AA. This feeds into our tendency to judge. We notice everything and there are lots of things that "bug" us about meetings.

Allowing clients to express their pet peeves without being judged themselves can be useful in breaking down the resistance, and in introducing the notion of tolerance toward others.

This group is short and simple and clients really enjoy it. It is a legitimate complaint session. Everyone gets to whine without feeling shamed or put down.

Group Discussion:

Today we are going to talk about meetings. We have heard both in AA/NA and in treatment that attending meetings is the single most important component to maintaining our sobriety. The recommendation is to attend 90 meetings in 90 days. This is a major commitment. Why do they suggest that anyway? It seems like overkill doesn't it?

The fact is that for most alcoholics and addicts, getting involved with new people in the program can be difficult and there are things about meetings that really ***"Bug the hell out of us."*** Ninety meetings in 90 days can help us move through these issues in early sobriety.

- How many people here like going to meetings?

- Who does not like meetings?

Whether you like meetings or not there are bound to be things that bother you about them. The size of meetings and all the different personalities are likely to set off pet peeves, and we often keep them to ourselves. Today we are going to give each other permission to tell the group what things "bug" us about meetings.

Generate a group list of complaints or criticisms.

Example:

What Bugs Me About AA Meetings:

1. People who repeat themselves.
2. People who talk too long.
3. Big Book thumpers.
4. Preachers
5. Advice Givers.
6. Noisy kids.
7. Smoking meetings.
8. Non-Smoking meetings.
9. People who distract (talk while another is talking).
10. People who get up for coffee.
11. Ego maniacs.
12. Pity potters.
13. Opinion givers.
14. Tear jerkers.
15. Uncomfortable chairs.
16. People who don't talk loud enough.
17. Foul language.
18. AA jargon.
19. People who give a drunkalog when they are not the speaker.
20. Holding hands.
21. Saying the Lord's Prayer.
22. No decaf coffee.
23. The meeting is too long.
24. Long winded announcements at the end of the meeting.
25. Drunks at meetings.

Considering all of the problems with meetings, how do we keep ourselves going? These concerns and complaints are not unusual. The founders of AA noted this problem early on. They even wrote a tradition about it. Tradition Twelve: *"Anonymity is the spiritual foundation of all our traditions, ever reminding us to place principles before personalities."*

- How do you deal with these things in your sobriety?
- What does "Principles before personalities" mean to you?
- What is your commitment to meetings?

Spend time with your clients reviewing each complaint and **the solutions.**

INTRODUCTION TO THE CODEPENDENCY GROUPS

Codependency has become an enormous field. It has not yet been recognized by the American Psychiatric Association as a separate disease process. This leaves much of the etiology and symptomatology of codependency open to discussion and interpretation.

Most treatment facilities do agree that if you scratch the surface of an addict/alcoholic, you will find a codependent. Many clinicians also believe that addiction is a **symptom** of codependency. They believe that the codependency initially develops during childhood. Chemical use becomes a way to relieve or cope with it, and that eventually the addiction takes on a life of its own and becomes the primary disease for those genetically predisposed to addiction. Once treated for addiction, the client still has unresolved, underlying codependency.

There are also different schools of thought complete with their own statistics about when and how to explain and resolve "codependency" issues. Some facilities begin codependency and abuse issues the day the client has detoxed. Others suggest that their clients have a year of sobriety before delving into their psyches.

It would be foolish for us to suggest the extent and intensity of the codependency you need to address in treatment. We do not know the types of clients you serve, your clinical skills, your ability to provide emotional safety for your client, or your treatment philosophy. However, since most alcoholics come from alcoholic or dysfunctional homes, most of them have significant codependency issues with relationships, intimacy, and self-esteem. Relapse rates are extremely high for individuals who do not have the skills to cope with these issues. It is within this context that we suggest laying an initial foundation so that your clients may cope with their emotional life after the chemicals are out of their bodies and they are thinking again. Since the term "codependency" works well within the treatment and recovering community, we choose to place these groups within that framework.

Our intention is not to teach the therapist about codependency. There are excellent resources and materials available to you at most bookstores. Rather, our goal is to show you the ways we have found to be very successful in presenting the available materials to your clients and their families.

The following lectures and groups are designed to help your clients understand the development of their "codependency." They are intended to provide a theoretical framework to assist your clients to see "why they are the way they are." Once your clients understand the general theory, they are then able to personalize it to fit their individual stories. With understanding comes illumination, then enlightenment.

As with the other presentations, there are wonderful materials available to you in bookstores and workshops. Use everything!

This is a series of groups and lectures **which is intended to be given in order.** It outlines the development of "codependency" or dysfunctional behavior.

CO-DEPENDENCY DISEASE CONCEPT LECTURE

This is an excellent introductory lecture to the concepts of codependency. Because it is a general introductory lecture, it avoids confrontation, denial, and resistance, while allowing your clients and families to begin to see themselves, "identify-in," and begin to understand the dynamics of their codependency.

This lecture can also be powerful for a mixed group of addicts and their significant others because it shows what they have in common. It is equally as powerful for a group consisting of addicts only. The lecture will validate their long-standing problems in relationships and provide hope for recovery in those areas.

Materials Needed: Blackboard

PART I : DEFINING ADDICTION:

1. To prepare for the group, write the following definition and table on the blackboard:

   Definition Of Addiction: A compulsive behavior with something external to ourselves, and continuing that behavior in spite of consequences to ourselves and/or others.

A **Disease Symptoms**	B **Disease Behaviors**	C **Feelings**
Preoccupation	Rationalizing	
Increased Tolerance	Minimizing	
Loss of Control	Blaming	
Denial	Euphoric Recall	
Delusion	Sneaking/Lying	
Blackouts	Hiding/Secrets	
Craving	Anger	
Compulsive Behavior	Shame	
Decreased Tolerance	Fear	
Frozen or "Numb" Feelings	Isolation	
Medical Problems		

Begin the group.

2. Ask for a show of hands from people who are:

    Chemically dependent
    Codependent
    Not sure

    Explain that after the group is completed, everybody will be sure about who they are.

3. After group introductions, inform the clients that the purpose of this group is to explain how the disease of codependency is nearly the same as the disease of addiction. Families will benefit if they understand that they have a very similar affliction as the addict. Very similar indeed.

    To see how codependency is a disease like addiction, we need to compare it to the disease of addiction.

4. Begin the lecture by reviewing the general definition of addiction on the blackboard. The "something external" in the definition can refer to alcohol, drugs, cigarettes, gambling, sex, food, etc.

5. Next, explain that you would like to review the **symptoms** and **behaviors** of addiction.

A **symptom** describes common characteristics of a disease. Coughing, high fever, high white blood cell count are symptoms of pneumonia or bronchitis. When we have a patient's symptoms, we can begin to diagnose the underlying disease. **Column A reviews symptoms of chemical dependency.**

When someone's body is affected by a disease, we expect them to show different **behaviors**. Sleeping, lethargy, poor appetite are the behaviors which accompany pneumonia. Addiction manifests with its own set of "classic" behaviors.

When reviewing the symptoms and behaviors, use group participation as much as possible. If your clients have had the lectures and groups on the Disease Concept and Denial, they should be able to practically run the group. This reinforces their knowledge of their disease.

> **For example,** beginning with "Disease Symptoms List," ask a group member, *"What is preoccupation? Give an example from your life."*

Help them with their definition verbally or write it on the board. Also, ask the family member to give examples of preoccupation for their addict in treatment. Mix it up.

6. Continue describing all of the items in both lists until they are complete.

A sample of how these completed lists might look is given below:

DISEASE SYMPTOMS:

Preoccupation = Thoughts about obtaining or using the chemical.

Example: "I wonder if there's enough booze at home, (or) if my dealer will be home, (or) if I have enough money for my chemicals."

Increased Tolerance = The ability to tolerate more and more of the chemical and achieve the same effect.

Example: "I used to get drunk on 6 beers. Now I can drink 8 beers."

Loss of Control = Inability to predict my using behavior. I may get drunk, I may not.

Example: "I only planned to have a glass of wine at the wedding. I got drunk and passed out."

Denial = A subconscious defense which tells us we do not have the disease.

Example: "Everybody drinks, don't they? It doesn't mean I'm alcoholic."

Delusion = A lie we tell ourselves which we truly believe.

Note: Explain to the group that there are levels to the severity of delusions. Some people have severe delusions. They truly believe that they are Napoleon or Jesus Christ. Alcoholics also have delusions, and they truly believe that they are telling the truth.

Example: "My children have not been affected by my drinking."

Blackouts = A period of amnesia.

Example: "I can't remember where I parked my car last night."

Craving = Physical need for the chemical.

Example: "I wanted cocaine so bad I could taste it."

Compulsive Behavior = Acting out behavior to reduce the craving or preoccupation.

Example: "When I had the craving, I knew I shouldn't drink, but I found myself in the bar last night anyway."

Frozen Or Numb Feelings = Limited range of feelings, difficult to feel too "high" or happy, too low or sad. Staying in gray emotional areas.

Example: "I heard a dear friend of mine was killed. I thought it was too bad, but that's life." "I haven't cried in two years."

Decreased Tolerance = The body breaks down, cannot drink or use as much without becoming drunk or sick.

Example: "Now, my speech gets slurred after one drink, and I get sick more often."

Medical Problems = When tolerance decreases, it is a sign of end stage addiction. (Refer to "Medical Consequences Lecture" for list of symptoms — liver disease, etc.)

After this section,

Ask the group: Does this make sense so far?
To the addicts: Did you see this in your disease?
To the codependents: Did you see this in your significant others?

Because of group time constraints, keep this section fairly simple. Allow about five minutes for discussion.

Having completed Column 4, continue the lecture by reviewing Column B. Do the same review with the Disease Behaviors List, asking the group for the definitions of terms and a personal example. Give examples of disease behavior and how we see them on the outside.

DISEASE BEHAVIORS:

Rationalizing = Making excuses about the using behavior.

Example: "I drank because I had a bad day."

Minimizing = Reducing the severity of the abuse.

Example: "A six pack of beer isn't much. I'm not that sick."

Blaming = Holding another person, place, or thing responsible for the using.

Example: "My husband makes me mad. If **he** didn't irritate me so much, I wouldn't need to use."

Euphoric Recall = Only remembering how good it felt, not how sick you got.

Example: "Ahh, there's nothing like *cocaine* or a *cold beer*."

Real Recall would be: "There's nothing like my cocaine paranoia, or puking my guts out after cold beer on my *alcoholic bleeding ulcer!*"

Sneaking/Lying = Being dishonest about the chemical use.

Example: "I told my boyfriend I was at the movies last night. I was really at the bar with my friends."

Hiding/Secrets = Not sharing the true extent of the problem, concealing the facts.

Example: "I keep an extra bottle in the trunk of my car."

Anger = Inability to cope with perceived injustices, judgments about what we can or cannot do, or defense mechanisms around other feelings, i.e., shame.

Example: "I blew up at my wife when she asked me not to drink."

Shame = Intense feeling of being "defective," "something's wrong with me."

Example: "I yelled at my wife yesterday and hurt her feelings. I had to go home drunk today. I couldn't face her."

Fear = State of apprehension resulting from perceived threat.

Example: "I was hungover and called in sick yesterday. I couldn't go back today. I didn't want my boss to say something to me."

Isolation = Decreased interaction with others. Lessened ability to be intimate or feel at ease with others.

Example: " I'd rather stay home and drink by myself."

When completed, ask the same questions to the group.
Does this make sense to you?
To the addicts: Do you see your behaviors in this list?
To the codependents: Do you see your significant others in the list?

Allow for a few minutes to share.

For column C, Feelings, ask the addicts to make a list of the feelings that they have while in their disease:

Sample:

Depressed
Sad
Alone
Ashamed
Angry, Etc.

Now for the fun part.
Explain that for some reason, many people think that our codependents have the same disease as the addict.

HOW CAN THAT BE?

PART II : DEFINING CODEPENDENCY

Go back to the blackboard.
Erase the word "addiction" from the blackboard.
Erase all of the examples you may have filled in, leaving only the original lists with the terms and feelings.
Replace the word addiction you have just erased with the word "codependent."
Explain that this is actually the definition for codependence.

It's only possible to get a codependent's attention by tricking them into believing that you're going to teach them more about their addicts. So that's what you just did. Apologize and tell them that this probably won't happen again!

1. Go through the two lists again with the focus this time on codependency. It is crucial that you focus each example with an **"I statement"** about **"my disease of codependency."** The focus of the family members will be to continue to see the disease of addiction. **Keep the focus on the codependent's disease.** If you, the therapist, are a codependent in recovery, use examples from your own history. Ask permission of the family members to use examples you see in them, or if they would like to volunteer their own examples.

(If the families are not present during this lecture, just the addicts, explain that this next section is what happens to their families.)

Since the definitions of the terms have already been explained, go through the lists with different examples for codependence.

A completed list of Disease Symptoms Examples in Column A, might look like this (heavily emphasizing the **"I" statements**):

DISEASE SYMPTOMS

Preoccupation: "**I am** preoccupied with where my husband is, who he is with, and what I will say to him."

Increased Tolerance: "**I have** increased tolerance to the dysfunction and the pain in the relationship."

Note — Increased tolerance is a good point to heavily stress: *"If somebody had told me when we got married, that 10 years later, I would be married to a drunk who lies constantly to me, who steals money from my purse, who ignores the kids, who expects me to make love to him drunk, who I can't talk to or feel close to, I would have run screaming from the altar. The fact that I have somehow ended up in this situation shows that I have increased tolerance to the pain."*

Loss of Control: "When **I know** that he is going to be late for dinner again, I usually give him the cold shoulder and go about my business. That's my plan. On occasion, I'll just snap. Yesterday, I was planning on ignoring him, but I ended up screaming *in front of the kids.* **I,** not my husband, **was out of control."**

Denial: **"I'm** not sick . He has the problem, not me. I haven't changed at all."

Delusion: "The kids have not been affected **by me** or **my behavior."**

Blackouts: "We had a screaming fight the other night. **I don't remember exactly what I** said."

Craving: "I really miss him. When he is gone, **my** whole body aches."

Compulsive Behavior: "I tell myself that I am not eating the chocolate cake. **I eat it** anyway." (Compulsive behaviors include workaholism, perfectionism, other addictive disorders.)

Frozen Or Numb Feelings: "I used to laugh a lot, and feel happy and carefree. **I haven't felt happy** and carefree in years."

Decreased Tolerance: **"I can't take** anymore. Everything he does irritates me."

Note — *Point out that decreased tolerance is usually what motivates the codependent to get help. It is an emotional bottom.*

Medical Problems: **"I have** constant headaches and high blood pressure."

Note: *If the codependent does not get help for themselves, they will have medical problems. Some will be fatal. Initial medical problems are headaches, muscle aches, fatigue, and depression.*

Serious end stage medical problems include **hypertension** (repressed anger leaves blood vessels in constant states of constriction, resulting in hypertension). Hypertension leads to **strokes** and **heart attacks. Eating disorders** and significant **emotional disorders** develop, particularly **major depression** which is life threatening. **Suicide** may be a danger if the codependent does not get help.

Ask the families if they can relate to this list and have them give examples.

2. Review the next list, **Column B,** Disease Behaviors, remembering to keep it focused on **my** dysfunction.

DISEASE BEHAVIORS

Rationalizing: "I make excuses about why I'm sleeping more or why I'm irritated. It's the weather or the kids."

Minimizing: "I didn't really lose control when I screamed in front of the kids. Maybe a little, but the kids have seen worse on TV."

Blaming: "It's his fault that I've changed. If **he would** quit drinking, I could be happy."

Euphoric Recall: "How can I leave him? It used to be so good. I remember our honeymoon, he was so sweet. I really love him."

Sneaking/Lying: "I told him the gas bill was $100. It was only $80. I told my mother we are doing fine. **I've** become a liar."

Hiding/Secrets: "I don't want to go to parties anymore. I don't want my friends to see us this way. I don't even tell the kids their Dad is an alcoholic."

Anger: "I wake up angry. **I'm** always mad at work or with the kids."

Shame: "If I was prettier, he wouldn't drink. **I'm** a terrible parent."

Fear: "Tell him he's an alcoholic? Tell the kids, my family and the boss that he's an alcoholic? No way. He could lose his job. My family will judge us. **I'm** afraid."

Isolation: "I don't go out with my friends anymore. I hardly have any friends. I can't tell anybody how I am really feeling. I feel all alone."

When the list is complete, continue with column C, Feelings. Ask the families how they feel in the feeling list. The feelings should be nearly identical to the list the addicts developed.

Can the group relate to this?
Can they give examples?
Ask the addicts to give examples of how their codependents do these behaviors?
Do they see that if they removed the word addiction from the picture, **they have the same disease?**

This is also a good time to show how both diseases are chronic, progressive, and fatal, manifested by tolerance and loss of control.

PART III.

Here's the third part of the magic act you have been performing.

1. Now, address the addicts again. Ask them to put their "chemical dependency" label on the shelf for the moment.

2. Ask them to remove their families from the list on the blackboard and **to substitute their own names.** Ask them to plug themselves back into the definition of codependency.

3. Go briefly through the list again with the addicts being the codependents. Do they see that when they are not using, they are also codependent? **Can they see how they experience these symptoms, behaviors, and feelings, especially when they're in relationships?**

- Before their addiction took on a life of its own, they did the codependency trip.
- They found something or someone outside of themselves to fix their insides.
- When they quit using, they will go back to their own pattern of codependency.
- After their craving for the drug leaves and they are able to stay sober, they will be working on their underlying codependency the same as anyone else.
- There is little difference between us as addicts or codependents, we're just people.
- We share the same disease.
- Our recovery will look the same.
- People are people.

PART IV : RECOVERY FROM CODEPENDENCY

Addicts are codependents.

Codependents are addicted to their codependency.

Going back to the chalkboard, draw a garbage can. **The use of metaphor works well for groups.**

Sample Metaphor:

We are like garbage cans coming into treatment, the addicts and the codependents alike. *As you review the following, label and explain the garbage can.*

- **The outsides are our defenses.** We're as tough as steel. Rocks bounce off us.

- **The inside is how we are really feeling,** the nasty garbage. Feelings of shame, anger, pain, fear of abandonment, loneliness, our secrets. All of this is tightly sealed in by the lid of the garbage can, festering.

Somewhere underneath all of this garbage is our self-worth, our ability to love, feel joy, and be creative. It is so mixed up with the garbage that **the whole thing smells bad.**

- The lid keeps our garbage inside. **The lid is our denial**— minimizing, rationalizing, blaming, intellectualizing, and so forth.

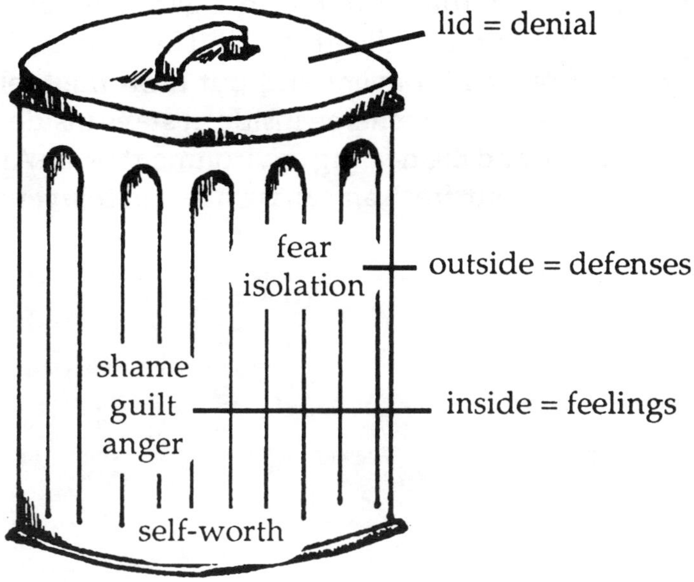

The only way to recover from any disease is to take the lid off and clean out the garbage.

The first step in doing this is to break through the defenses and the denial about how sick we are.

This is the first step in Al-Anon or Codependent's Anonymous — to recognize that I'm powerless over__________, and that my life is unmanageable.

Nobody held a gun to my head and said "go through his wallet" or "sneak around and check up on him" or "scream in front of the kids." There was no gun to my head. I developed this **all on my own.** **<u>My</u>** life is unmanageable, **<u>I'm</u>** out of control.

Note: The therapist really needs to stress the above message. The codependents in the group initially have an *impossible* time understanding how *they* have the problem. Use 10 to 20,000 examples of how the **codependent** becomes "unmanageable." **I'm** depressed, **I'm** angry, **I'm** mean to the kids, **my** feelings are out of control.

The first step is breaking through my denial.

I'm powerless and I'm sick. I'm done with denial!

The second step is getting the garbage out. **This is an action step!** Thinking about garbage and simply recognizing it is not the solution. If I see garbage in a trash can and sit around thinking about it, **the garbage is still in the trash can.**

Taking the trash out, means taking the trash out! It means taking out each secret and exposing it to air. Nasty rotting things in a garbage can ,when exposed to air, will quit rotting, dry up, and eventually disintegrate. The fresh air is the spirituality in Al-Anon. I take out my secret or painful event and put it on the table. This is Al-Anon or family therapy. If I leave the secret or shame inside, it stays inside. If I put it on the table, it is not inside of me anymore and the healing environment of Al-Anon and others can help heal it. When I get my garbage out, fresh air can rush in and rejuvenate my joy, love, and creativity.

Recovery is:

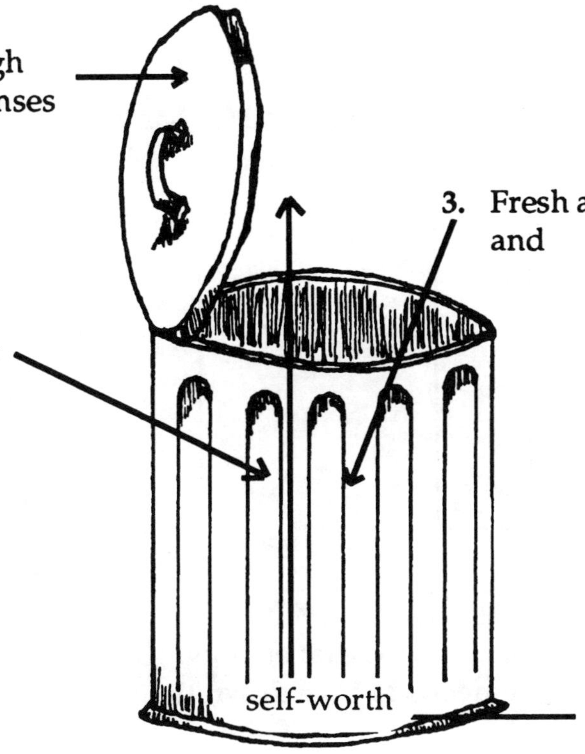

A second use of metaphor also helps to reinforce the concept. A metaphor which is really gross but everybody can relate to is that of a wound.

Codependence is like having a festering wound on your arm. It is not going away. You don't know how to fix it so you put a bandage on top of it. This is what we were taught in dysfunctional families. Cover it up.

The wound gets worse and worse. It gets really gross and filled with pus and we keep the bandages on. The wound is our internal wound, the bandage is our denial and way to protect our wound.

The therapist or doctor tells us that the only way to clean the wound is to take the bandage off, clean out the pus which is painful, and expose the wound to air or Al-Anon.

We have two choices. We can do nothing, leave the bandage on, and lose the arm.

We can clean out the cut, let fresh blood came to the surface and expose it to air.
(For borderline or horrifically abused patients, metaphors around a huge wound and only debriding a part of it at a time are helpful here.)

A final example **WHEW!!! WE'RE DOWN THE HOME STRETCH NOW!!!** is to draw two stick figures with two walls between them.

Having done the exercise, we know that we're all the same at a feeling level and with our defenses.

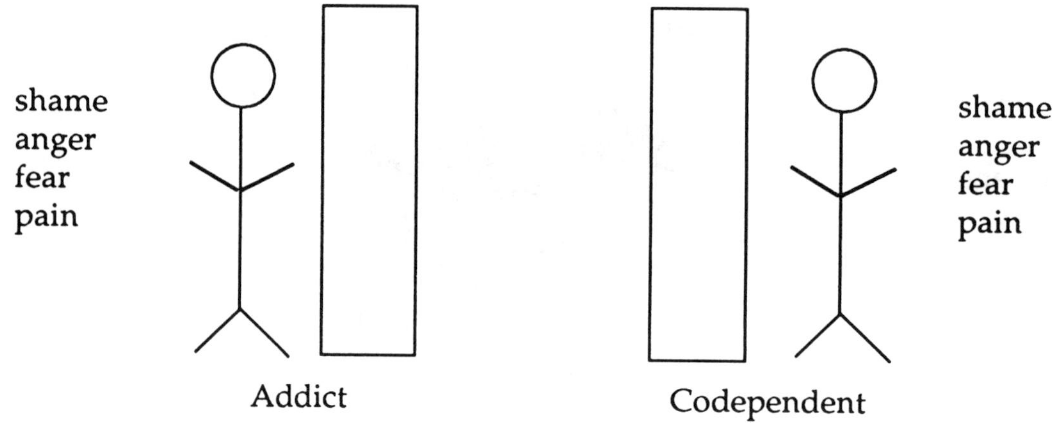

To heal the relationship the wall needs to be taken down, brick by brick. **Since each person created their wall, each person needs to take down their wall.**

When the wall or denial comes down, our feelings and our vulnerability are exposed. **This is the work in therapy and 12 Step meetings - Being real and honest about our vulnerability and feelings so we can transform them.**

Demonstrate this:

Erase the addict's wall and their feelings from the diagram.
If only the addict is doing the work, what does the relationship look like?
All parties need to work their own program.

Erase the second wall. Erase the word "shame."
If I only talk about my shame, what is still left in the relationship?
My anger, fear and pain are still present, alive and festering.

PART V : CLOSING THE GROUP

Ask the group for feedback about what they heard.
What did they particularly relate to?
Did it make sense to them? Which parts?

Does each person understand that to recover, they each need to take the walls down and work on their own feelings?

To recover, they will need to begin to make decisions about being willing to do their own work, work their own program.

Will they start looking at their denial, bring it to group and talk about it? Will they take out the garbage?

Will they start going to Al-Anon or be part of the problem?

Ask for a show of hands of people who now realize that they are codependents.

Congratulate them and welcome them to the program of emotional sobriety!!!

CODEPENDENT BEHAVIOR

This group is written as a follow-up to **Codependency Disease Concept.**

Materials: Blackboard

Objectives :

1. Clients will identify specific codependent behavior.
2. Clients will understand the need for their own recovery.

There are many definitions of codependency. The definition used here is from "Codependent No More," by Melody Beattie. "A codependent is a person who has let someone else's behavior affect him or her and is obsessed with controlling other people's behavior."

As codependents we have been so focused on the problems of the alcoholic, that to suddenly shift the focus to ourselves can be uncomfortable and threatening. If we are alcoholic, our codependency has been very tied into the coping mechanisms and defenses of our own alcoholism. "Putting the plug in the jug" will not make our problems in relationships magically disappear.

We thought our problem was solved when the alcoholic finally became willing to get help and stop drinking. Now, these people are telling me that I'm sick too and need to recover! We had no idea that this was part of the bargain.

Remember that no one here caused alcoholism, but all of us have been affected by it. That is what we will be exploring in this group.

As codependents we all suffered injury to self-esteem. It would be harmful to use this information to torture ourselves. The fact is that the motivation for our behavior and interactions, more often than not, was out of caring, concern, and a desire to help. We made choices and reviewed the options available at the time.

A typical codependent's response to new insight and awareness about the disease concept is to do a litany of "If only's..."

For example: *"If only I didn't pay his rent the last six months, maybe he would have sought help sooner."*

"If only's" and **"I should haves"** are not allowed. We did the best we could with what we had and that is good enough. We cannot take our understanding and time travel to change the past. **Our responsibility lies in response to knowledge that we have today.**

We have developed behavior habits, responses, and reactions to others. In recovery, some of those need to change. Change requires practice. We do not make these changes overnight. We will explore three of the most common codependent behaviors, **enabling, caretaking** and **controlling.**

1. Enabling: Enabling is behavior which protects or prevents another person from experiencing the consequences of his own behavior.

This can be most obvious in our relationship with the alcoholic but also occurs in our other relationships. **There are two problems with enabling:**

> The first problem is that if there are no negative consequences to the disease behavior, then there is no reason to change it.
>
> The second problem is that the person in trouble comes to depend on rescue from others instead of changing the problem.

As the disease of alcoholism progresses, it affects finances, marriages, relationships with children, work, etc. There may also be run-ins with the law and physical and mental illnesses. These are some of the areas that move us into protective or enabling behaviors.

Example: *"My wife has a hangover. She really laid one on last night. She will never make it to work today. I will call her boss and tell him she has a virus. I will have to make up symptoms so he doesn't suspect it has to do with drinking and fire her."*

I have protected my wife's job and protected her alcoholism by lying to her boss. After all, "she needs the job and I wouldn't want anyone to know that she drinks too much."

Using the blackboard, have the group **generate a list** of enabling behaviors which they have used to protect someone from facing consequences. Add a second column labeled **cost to me and others.** Add a third column labeled **help or hindrance?**

Spend some time with the group completing and discussing all three columns.

2. Caretaking: When one person takes on the responsibility of another.

Caretaking inhibits the other person from adequately caring for himself. It affects the other's ability to grow and function as an adult. It falsely boosts the self-esteem of the codependent, who feels needed.

This behavior also creates inequality and lack of balance in adult relationships. An example of this is found in the relationship category of responsibility. By caretaking, one person is **overly responsible** which allows the other person to be **under responsible.**

Example: *"I am a nurse. My sister needs to make her first doctor's appointment. She calls and is feeling a little anxious about the call. To relieve her anxiety, I make the appointment for her. For the next five years, I make all the phone calls related to health care for my sister, her husband and her two children. She has developed irrational fear and significant anxiety about this issue and feels unable to do it on her own. At first I was glad to help. Now, I'm tired of this and resentful."*

Is this a help or a hindrance?

Make a second list of the group's caretaking behaviors. Add a second list about what it cost them and others when they acted as caretaker. Did it help?

3. **Controlling:** Controlling behaviors are those we use to force a desired outcome.

We live in an "out of control" environment with people who are unpredictable and unreliable at best. We take matters into our own hands to "keep things together" and to maintain our sanity.

The goal of control is to make you do what I want you to do according to my beliefs and values. It does not allow others to make their own decision. It induces shame and guilt and judgment. Most of us learned this behavior in our family of origin.

To recover we must begin to let go of our control over others, and to focus on ourselves. *"I cannot do my work if I am busy doing yours."*

Example: *"I am in treatment and my wife has just had the lecture on the recovery process. She heard that if an alcoholic follows the recovery suggestions that sobriety is a guarantee. She thinks, "Hmmm, I can help with this one! Since Joe lost his license because of that last DWI, I'll just rearrange my work schedule so I can take him to meetings. I could even go with him to make sure he doesn't leave. The sponsor thing is no problem. My friend Mary's husband goes to AA. I'll call her tonight to arrange it. Now, Joe needs to meditate, so I'll stop by the bookstore on the way home and pick up a few meditation books. If I find he's not reading that "Big Book", I'll just set it by his TV chair and remind him. This is terrific!* ***I just know my Joe will stay sober!"***

There are a whole host of behaviors we use to attempt control. Here are just a few:

Nagging
Demanding
Placating
Complaining
Supervising
Lecturing
Hollering
Playing the victim
Whining
Commanding
Trying to make others feel guilty
Threatening to hurt ourselves or someone else
Using sex as punishment or reward
Threatening to have a heart attack

There are reasons and benefits for us in controlling behavior.

- What are some of the situations you have tried to control?
- Why do you try to control?

Examples: *" I think I have to. "*
" I'm trying to help."

What are the benefits to us when we are in charge?

Examples: *"It takes away pain."*
"It feels like a loving thing to do."
"It reinforces that I know best."
"I get to be right."
"It gives me a sense of power."
"They need me."

Generate a list of control behaviors from the group and the consequences of their controlling behavior. Did it help?

Ask them to identify a favorite controlling behavior.

The beginning of recovery is the recognition that my behavior is not working for me or for those I love. This can give us the impetus we need to grow and change and to work a program of recovery. Letting go of control is not easy. Help is available in Al-Anon, Adult Children of Alcoholics and Codependents Anonymous.

Each person must work his own program.

Going to meetings together is not recommended. Concerns over the way another person is working recovery can move us back into control mode. Bring concerns to your sponsor and to meetings, where you can get the help you need to refocus on your own recovery.

The road to recovery is rewarding. We can achieve balance and health in our relationships with others.

There is a wealth of self-help literature available to assist in dealing with codependency.

HANDOUTS: Reading resource list and Al-Anon check list. You may also want to hand out a copy of the area Al-Anon schedule.

Do a separate follow up group with the family. Review the Al-Anon list. Discuss each question:

- How is this a symptom of codependency and why?
- Is Al-Anon for you?
- What is your resistance to attending Al-Anon?

Use this group to answer family questions about Al-Anon, addressing concerns, and myths.

See the lecture "Twenty Questions" to use as a simple guide.

HANDOUT #37

READING RESOURCE LIST

Melody Beattie,	*Codependent No More*
Melody Beattie,	*Beyond Codependency*
Robert Becker, PhD.,	*Addicted to Misery. The Other Side of Codependency*
Claudia Black,	*It Will Never Happen To Me*
John Bradshaw,	*The Family*
Colette Dowling,	*The Cinderella Complex - Women's Hidden Fear Independence*
Ernie Larson,	*Stage II Recovery: Life Beyond Addiction*
Pia Mellody,	*Facing Codependence*
Robin Norwood,	*Women Who Love Too Much*
M. Scott Peck, M.D.,	*The Road Less Traveled*
Theodore Rubin,	*The Angry Book*
Anne Wilson Schaeff,	*Codependence, Misunderstood - Mistreated*
Robert Subby,	*Lost in the Shuffle: The Codependent Reality*
Janet Geringer Woititz Ed,D.,	*Adult Children of Alcoholics*
C.L. Whitfield,	*Healing the Child Within*

HANDOUT #38

Al-Anon: IS IT FOR YOU?

Millions of people are affected by the excessive drinking of someone close. The following questions are designed to help you decide whether or not you need Al-Anon.

		Yes	No
1.	Do you worry about how much someone else drinks?	____	____
2.	Do you have money problems because of someone else's drinking?	____	____
3.	Do you tell lies to cover up for someone else's drinking?	____	____
4.	Do you feel that drinking is more important to your loved one than you are?	____	____
5.	Do you think that the drinker's behavior is caused by his or her companions?	____	____
6.	Are mealtimes often delayed because of the drinker?	____	____
7.	Do you make threats, such as "if you don't stop drinking I will leave you"?	____	____
8.	When you kiss the drinker hello, do you secretly try to smell his or her breath?	____	____
9.	Are you afraid to upset someone for fear it will set off a drinking bout?	____	____
10.	Have you been hurt or embarrassed by a drinker's behavior?	____	____
11.	Does it seem as if every holiday is spoiled because of drinking?	____	____
12.	Have you considered calling the police because of drinking behavior?	____	____

	Yes	No
13. Do you find yourself searching for hidden liquor?	____	____
14. Do you feel that if the drinker loved you, he or she would stop drinking to please you?	____	____
15. Have you refused social invitations out of fear or anxiety?	____	____
16. Do you sometimes feel guilty when you think of the lengths you have gone to control your drinker?	____	____
17. Do you think that if the drinker stopped drinking your other problems would be solved?	____	____
18. Do you ever threaten to hurt yourself to scare the drinker into saying "I'm sorry" or "I love you"?	____	____
19. Do you ever treat people (children, employees, parents, co-workers) unjustly because you are angry at someone else for drinking too much?	____	____
20. Do you feel there is no one who understands your problems?	____	____

If you answered yes to three or more of these questions, Al-Anon or Alateen may help.

DYSFUNCTIONAL FAMILIES

Some of our clients already know that they come from dysfunctional families while others are hard pressed to believe it. By giving a presentation of an overall view of functional versus dysfunctional families to start, you can avoid power struggles and begin to illuminate your clients.

Materials Needed: Blackboard

Start this group by informing the members that it is suggested that **all** alcoholics/addicts come from dysfunctional families. (That ought to rattle them!)

It is believed that 96 percent of families in the United States are dysfunctional. HOW CAN THIS BE?

Some symptoms of our dysfunctional society are:

1. We have the highest addiction rate of any country in the world.

2. We use more addicting prescription drugs of any country in the world.

We are among the top ten countries in:

1. Mental illness.

2. Violence and violent crime.

3. Suicide and suicide in **children**.

How we've been raised in families is not working! These groups are not about finding blame. They are simply about looking at the system to see what is not working so it can be changed.

Notes To The Clinician: It is imperative with all of these groups, that you ask clients to look at their own family systems as **they** were growing up. There is often a tendency for patients who are parents to want to see how they have affected their kids. To recover, they first need to identify and feel **what happened to them.** Continuing to look at their parent's or their children's lives is a way for them to subconsciously keep their denial, avoid their pain, and stay out of recovery. Recovery is completely dependent on their ability to own **their** truth. Identifying with another person veils the abuse and allows them to avoid their own work.

A dysfunctional family is simply defined as a family where one or more of the individuals are not having their needs met. Brainstorm with the group about what is meant by this. What are the needs of all children?

Start a list on the blackboard making certain it is fairly complete.

Children's needs (include the concepts of):

Unconditional love
Acceptance
Trust (including issues about abandonment and betrayal)
Respect and recognition
Being listened to
Creativity/spontaneity
Touch

Pose these questions to the group:

1. If the child is told that he is loved but is rarely touched, what happens to the child? Ask similar questions related to the above list eliminating one of the needs and asking "What happens to the child who is not **accepted**, has not experienced **trust**, etc.?"

2. Who is responsible for creating this environment? Is the child responsible? No, parents are **completely** responsible for creating this environment. Emphasize this fact.

When all of the ingredients of the child's needs are present, the child has the opportunity to develop into a whole or completely functional human being. When some of the ingredients are missing, the family is dysfunctional. They are not functioning to meet all of the needs of the child and the child becomes impaired — they do not trust, or they do not know they are important, etc.

Families develop rules or sets of behaviors and expectations which are either functional (meet all the needs of the child and family) or dysfunctional (do not meet all the needs of the child and family).

On the blackboard, set up two columns:

DYSFUNCTIONAL	**FUNCTIONAL**

Have the group brainstorm about the "family rules" they know are dysfunctional, i.e., "big boys don't cry," and to identify the corresponding functional system, ie., "all feeings are acceptable."

DYSFUNCTIONAL	**FUNCTIONAL**
Big boys don't cry.	All feelings are acceptable.

Depending upon whichever "Adult Children" resource you prefer, spend most of the group setting up the two lists. Add, modify, and explain the categories. Have the list be as specific as possible and be certain that you confront myths. **For example:** With the rule, "big boys don't cry" (a common theme), ask them to be more specific and also challenge the rule. *"So, big boys don't cry. How old is a big boy, one-year old? Is a big boy three-years old? So, at what age should a `big boy' stop crying? What if their mom dies? What if the child is hit by mom, a brother, or a rock? Why aren't they supposed to cry?* ***What does crying mean?*** *This all sounds pretty crazy."* In a functional family, what is the goal? (All people are allowed to feel and share their pain.)

Many people have written different theories and various examples of dysfunctional family rules. Again, use them all or examples from your own life.

In general, these concepts of functional family systems need to be discussed:

Unconditional love and respect
Self-worth
Self-expression and individuality
Creativity
Expression of all feelings and ideas

While doing this group, remind the clients that most of our rules are learned from our parents who learned the rules from their parents, etc. This means that dysfunctional families **are generational**, and like alcoholism, *if left untreated, will become more severe in the ensuing generations.*

Ask the group to give specific examples from their own childhood. Some ideas to process are:

DYSFUNCTIONAL	VS	FUNCTIONAL
Conditional love: **Example:** *"I love you if you are 'good', get straight A's, are nice to your sister, etc."*	**VS**	**Unconditional love:** **Example:** *"I love you completely."* Here, the parent is able to separate the child from their destructive behaviors. "I love you and you cannot hit your sister vs **you're** bad for hitting her."
Secrets: Dysfunctional families have family secrets which are not talked about. Have the group list some secrets, i.e., divorces, illegitimate children, homosexuality, mental illness, financial ruin. *Secret keeping leads to shame or isolation — give examples.*	**VS**	**Open:** All things can be shared or discussed when age appropriate.
No boundaries or rigid boundaries: **No boundaries example:** Kids can't close bedroom or bathroom doors, can't tell somebody not to touch them, have to share private thoughts with somebody. **Rigid boundaries example:** **Example:** No touching or holding.	**VS**	**Healthy boundaries:** Privacy is respected, the child's body belongs to the child.
Punishment	**VS**	**Natural consequences**
Denial/Delusion: **Example:** *"Nothing's wrong. Things will get better."*	**VS**	**Truth and reality:** **Example:** Identifying and working through problems.
Blame: **Example:** *"You make me feel _____________."*	**VS**	**Responsibility:** **Example:** *"I feel ________." "I can __________."*
Indirect communication: **Example:** Triangulation: *"Tell your mother that I said ________."*	**VS**	**Direct Communication:** **Example:** Open communication and confrontation.
Rules: Rigid or separate for different family members.	**VS**	**Guidelines and flexibility**

Expectations: **Example:** All of the kids in this family get straight A's.	**VS**	**Individualism and self-worth**
Repression of certain feelings: **Example:** Anger, shame, love, fear.	**VS**	**All feelings shared, intimacy**
Suspicion	**VS**	**Trust**
Control	**VS**	**Creativity/Spontaneity**

When the list is exhausted, add a third column "Feelings and consequences to the child" to the left of the first two columns as follows:

Feelings & Consequences To The Child	**DYSFUNCTIONAL**	**FUNCTIONAL**
Shame, self loathing	**Conditional Love**	**Unconditional Love**

Have the group brainstorm about:

1. What the possible feelings are that the child would develop in this system. **Example:** If exposed to conditional love, would she feel shame, anger, etc.

2. How the child would be impaired as a result of the dysfunction. **Example:** Inability to trust, express anger, etc.

Go back through the entire list.
When completed, circle the "Feelings And Consequences" list. Inform the group that these are symptoms of having been in a dysfunctional family system.

Obviously, there are levels of severity of the dysfunction and the impairment created. However, it is important to show that children who **only have <u>some</u> of the symptoms still did not get their needs met. They grew up in a dysfunctional family.**

As therapists, many of us want our groups to end on a happy or positive note. This is a symptom of our codependency and our need to control the feelings of others. Needing "happy groups" is, if you will, a symptom of our own narcissism and emotional insecurity. These are difficult groups and only effective if the client can break through their denial to the pain underneath.

The first step in recovery is to break through denial (the garbage can theory). Here are some truths:

- We did not have completely perfect or wonderful childhoods.
- We are killing ourselves with numbing anesthetics.
- **Something was painful.**
- We did not learn how to tolerate pain and work through problems step by step.

This is the end of Part One on dysfunctional families. Most of your clients are now illuminated and "warmed up." There must be a follow-up group so they can share what they are remembering and the connections being made.

Follow-up Group

The follow-up group needs to correspond to those issues that came up for the clients during the lecture. The handout gives them the individual time they need for expressing these issues.

Pass out Handout #39, Dysfunctional Family Rules and:

1. Allow the group time to fill in their responses and then reconvene.

2. Allow each member to read their lists.

3. Give feedback. Be careful with the types of feedback allowed. Since your clients are "good codependents," they will want to make each other "feel good." *They will fall into the trap of dysfunctional family rule #1: "Don't feel bad. Everything is going to be okay. I am going to make sure I tell you that because I cannot tolerate your pain."* **Keep feedback limited to validating each other's experiences.** Example of feedback: *"When I heard you share your list I felt ________ or "That sounded scary to me."*

Close the group with a hand held circle to bring the group isolates back into the fold.

1. Remind the group that the exercise was not about blaming but about owning our truths.

2. Ask them to honor the children they were in those families.

3. Ask them to see each other as they are now, honest, feeling, remembering, and willing to recover.

HANDOUT #39

MY DYSFUNCTIONAL FAMILY RULES

Below, spend some time describing the ways in which you were raised with dysfunctional family rules. Please give one example of the rule as it applies to you. In Column B, give your impression of how you felt and some of the beliefs you developed about yourself. **Give examples:**

	A. Dysfunctional Family Rule:	B. Feelings & Resulting Beliefs:
1.		
2.		
3.		
4.		
5.		
6.		
7.		
8.		
9.		
10.		

ABOUT BLAME

When clients begin to work through their denial about not having perfect parents or perfect childhoods, they will generally respond with anger. Usually this anger takes on the form of blaming their parents for their current dysfunction.

There are two things about blame which are important to remember:

1. **Blame as a defense is a symptom of codependency.** Our clients grew up with blaming models. Blame works for people who don't know how or don't want to assume responsibility for their own actions. Blame also works as a defense against the underlying feelings of grief or abandonment repressed as a child.

2. Blame is a legitimate defense. In most cases, our clients did experience forms of abuse.

The problem lies in how to work with clients while they are in the "blame mode".

It is always recommended that you validate the clients' feelings. Not validating their feelings simply continues their abuse history of having their realities suppressed. Many therapists inadvertently steer their clients away from their underlying anger and blame. **This is a form of abuse.** Validating their feelings is of high priority. **For example:** *"I see your anger and I hear you blaming your parents. Am I correct? Can we explore this?"*

Sometimes explaining the following process to the client is helpful.

1. Assess whether the abuse of the family was **intentionally cruel.**

Intentional abuse by parents to children exists. Cruel people exist. If the abuse was obviously cruel or inhumane, validate this for the client. Refocus them on their primary goal of getting sober. The reason for this is that for the client to deal with their abuse issues, they will need sobriety, ego strengths, and different coping skills. During their first few weeks or months in treatment, they will have none of these skills. Focusing them on getting sober first will help them develop the coping skills they will later need to explore their abuse.

The way this looks is: *"John, I see that you are angry because your father used to whip you until you bled. You describe a brutal and traumatic childhood for which your father was responsible. I just wonder if you can stay sober now that you are beginning to have these memories and feelings?"*

Note: Unless you are a center which specializes in anger and rage integration work, acknowledge their reality of the abuse as it arises, while focusing them on the need to develop sobriety skills first. Include anger work or family therapy in their discharge planning to facilitate these issues with the specialists.

2. Assess if the abuse was **"not intentional"**, or covert abuse.

As clinicians, we believe that **ALL ABUSE IS ABUSE**. However, clients in early recovery usually need to protect their parents and repress their feelings. This is evident in their need to categorize levels, severity, and "intent" of the abuse.

If the client believes that the abuse was "not intentional", or covert, still acknowledge their feelings and memories. Explore the nature of the abuse and the intention of the parent. If the client feels that the abuse was not intentional, validate this as well. **For example:** *"John, I see how painful it is for you to remember how your mom was passed out drunk when you were little.* ***I'm glad you recognize this as abuse because it was abuse.*** *I also hear you say that you recognize that she did not set out to abuse you. How can you stay sober and reconcile these feelings for now?"* In this case, John's abuse issues have been heard and validated. The client also acknowledges the primary goal for developing tools for sobriety. There is also a clear implication for future work with these covert abuse issues.

****** It is important that the client understand that you are not asking or expecting them to forgive the abuses as this will only perpetuate their abuses. ******

For them to fully recover and achieve self-worth and intimacy, they will at some point need to work through their childhood issues. If you are not a facility which specializes in childhood abuse, you need to recognize and validate their feelings, perceptions, and experiences, while focusing them on the need to be able to stay sober in order to work through their issues.

In all cases of abuse and blame, the client must also be willing to be responsible for their current behaviors and relationships despite their histories. Recovery means being responsible for who they are today. When blaming the parents slip into their dynamic, they need to be refocused on assuming responsibility and control for their present situation. For Example: *"John, I hear you say that you hit your children as a punishment because that's how you were raised. Blaming your parenting skills on your upbringing may have been okay to explain your past behaviors. While these issues still need to be explored,*

Who will be responsible today if you hit them again?"

When I blame you legitimately or illegitimately, I am a victim. **Victim** pathology includes the dynamic of being helpless, passive, and under-responsible. Reframing blame statements (under-responsibility) with *"Who is responsible today?"* helps your clients stay out of their victim role in their present. It also empowers them to be able to take responsibility in exploring having been a victim.

For further explanation, refer to the "Abuse Triangle".

FAMILY ROLES

Introduction:

Families which are dysfunctional create family roles. It is important to remind your group of these things:

1. **Dysfunctional families usually don't know they are dysfunctional.** Nobody taught this subject in schools 20 or 100 years ago. These families are simply trying to do the best they can with what they have. When young people decide to have children, they don't do it so they can torture a tiny person. As children, we need to identify with and accept our parents, or suffer perceived abandonment. To confront abuse is inconceivable, so the child "identifies" with their parents and represses any thoughts, memories, or feelings of neglect or abuse. In order to survive, the child also accepts the dysfunctional rule, accepts the parent and copes. Now that the child sees the dysfunction as "normal", it is passed on to the next generation — *"It worked for me, didn't it?"*

   The response is simply, *"I don't know, you're in treatment aren't you? Did it* ***really*** *work for you?"*

2. **Dysfunctional families don't realize that they are creating family roles.** Again, role assignment is a subconscious process which evolves in a dysfunctional system.

   Because most of our parents were young and not completely mature at the time of our birth, they were usually unable to adequately relate to the child the difference existing between the child and the child's behavior. **For example:** Tommy spills the milk, mother is unhappy. It's the tenth time that it has happened today. **What Tommy internalizes** is that **Tommy** is bad, not that spilling the milk is the reason that mother is unhappy. It takes a particularly skillful mother to help Tommy see this difference. *The young, emotionally immature parent is unaware that this dynamic exists at all.* Tommy's behavior is frustrating to her. Tommy is **bad.** If Tommy is bad, the child who **does not** spill the milk is the **good** child. Now we have two family roles or labels, **the good child and the bad child.**

   Once the child is labeled, he is plugged into a subconscious role. Since Tommy has become the "bad" child, Mother does not take notice when he doesn't spill the milk, only when he does, so Tommy continues to get negative attention and fulfill his role. The second child gets the positive attention for not spilling. Negative attention is better than no attention and Tommy reinforces his role. This is obviously an oversimplification, but it works well with clients in early recovery.

3. **Family roles are assigned by the parents.** Usually, but not always, the first child is the good child (unless they were unwanted). By the time the second child is born, the first child is off and running and into trouble. So the new baby will become the "good baby" and the eldest will become "trouble".

   Each family is different depending upon the parents' emotional health. Some parents cope better with older children than with babies, so the babies are "trouble". It doesn't matter. The point is that the family role is created and given to your clients as children who were just being children.

4. **Family roles are interchangeable and shift over time.** The "good" child in first grade may begin to experience difficulty in eighth grade. He then becomes the "bad" child as the other child looks "good" in comparison. When he is in 12th grade, it may shift again and so forth. In any case, once the child is labeled, he also assumes the stereotypes of the label projected onto him by the parent.

   It is important that your clients understand that because they grew up in dysfunctional families, *roles were assigned to them.* These roles shifted over time as the family became more dysfunctional. **Because roles and labels are rigid, the child did not have the opportunity to discover their true nature and relationship to the world.**

5. **Most families have family roles.** The rigidity and consequences to the child assigned to that role varies depending upon the level of dysfunction in the family. In some families, the identified "bad" child may be "bad" throughout their history with that family. Other, less severely dysfunctional families may show flexibility in the roles as the parents mature.

The goal of this group is to allow your clients:

1. To identify their family roles.
2. Understand how their role affected them in the past and present.
3. Inspire and challenge new dimensions to their personal identities.

There is a lot of material available which goes into greater depth about family roles. Most of this material is found under the Adult Children Of Alcoholic modules. Familiarize yourself with this material, as well as with the various common definitions in your recovery community. Different therapists use different labels to describe similar behaviors. Inform your clients about your resources so they have an opportunity to explore these issues after treatment. **For example:** John Bradshaw and Claudia Black both have wonderful and informative material, however, their terms are different. The family hero, social worker, caretaker, enabler, and rescuer are all different labels describing similar roles by different sources. Choose one form which will best work for your setting.

For convenience sake, we will use these terms as developed by Sharon Wegscheider-Cruse and John Bradshaw:

Hero
Scapegoat
Lost Child
Mascot

Materials needed: Blackboard, writing pads, plain sheet of paper, Handout.

Reframe the information provided in the introduction to explain the need and goals for this group. Essentially, the purpose of the group is to allow the clients to begin to identify the roles assigned to their family and to them in the past, and to identify how these roles affect them in the present.

1. To begin, place large circles on the blackboard:

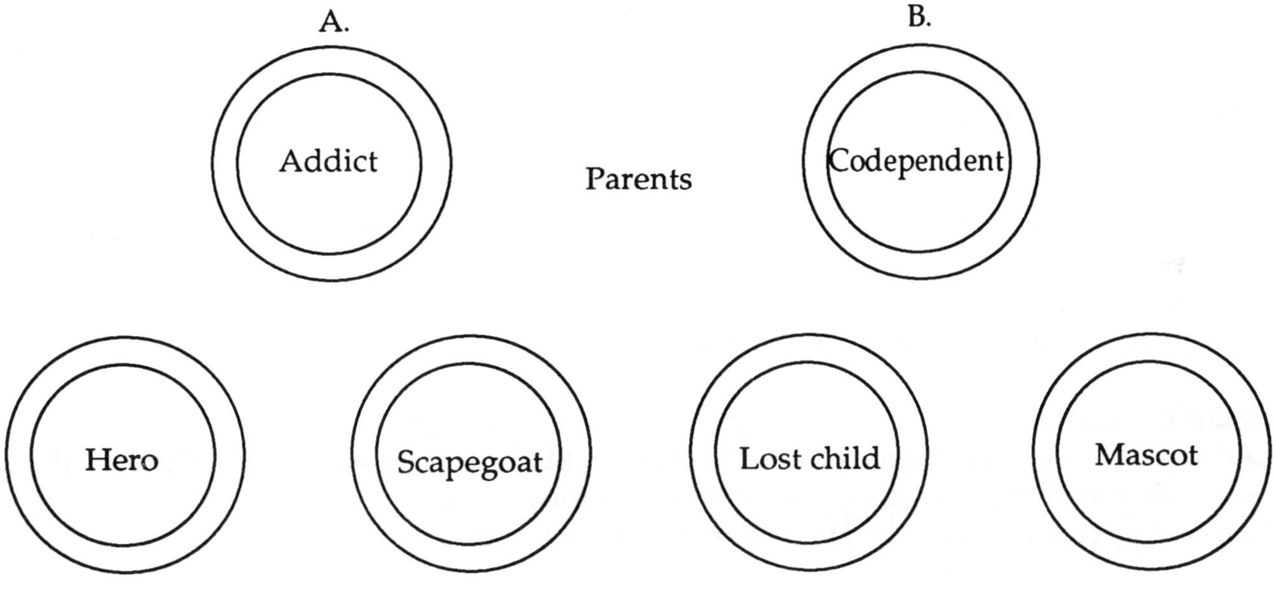

Circles A and B represent the parents.
One parent is usually the codependent, (enabler, rescuer, etc.) If the other parent is an addict, fill in the addict circle, otherwise leave blank for now.

The circles have two levels to them:
The **outer circle** identifies outside behaviors and defenses.
The **inner circle** identifies the inside, secret feelings.

2. Brainstorm with the group about completing the circles. **For example:** Using the Hero model, ask the group about outside behaviors. How does a family Hero look on the outside? In the family and at school?

Place these descriptions within the outside circle:

Family Hero:
Outside Behaviors: Overachiever, straight A's, surrogate parent, "good", perfectionist.
Outside Feelings: Happy, cheerful, in control.

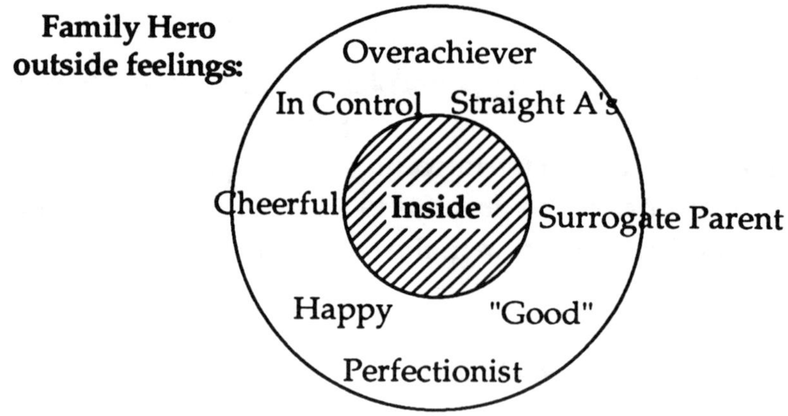

Can anybody in the group relate to this role?

3. Brainstorm about how this person feels on the inside, secretly: **For example: Inside Feelings:** Lonely, hurt, under confident, afraid.

Now place these descriptions on the inside circle.

Sample: Family Hero
Outside Appearance: Cheerful, Over Achiever, In Control, Straight A's, Cheerleader, Perfectionist, Surrogate Parent, Good, Happy
Inside Appearance: Lonely, Hurt, Under Confident, Afraid

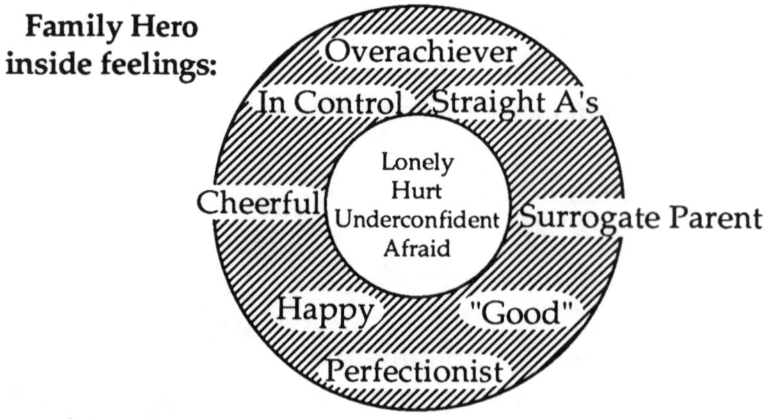

Who can relate to this role?

4. Do this with all of the roles. Complete all of the circles with the group. If you are going to use this model, include things like:

Sample: Scapegoat
Outside Appearance: "Bad", Defiant, Fights, Angry, Destructive, Self-Destructive, Negative Attention, Lying, Stealing, Etc.
Inside Appearance: Lonely, Worthless, Angry, Hurt, Abandoned, Sad

Sample: Lost Child
Outside Appearance: Withdrawn, Isolated, Loner, Few Friends, Plays By Self, Confused, Shy, Fantasy Life, Reads A Lot, Left Behind
Inside Appearance: Worthless, Lonely, Sad

Sample: Mascot
Outside Appearance: Clown, Joking, Stories (breaks up the tension in the family), Immature, Irresponsible, Pesty, Annoying, Family Pet
Inside Appearance: Fear (comes from feeling the tension in the family), Sadness, Confusion

Spend most of the group developing these models.

5. Toward the end of the group, have a group member copy the illustrated models from the board onto the plain paper. Make copies of this for a group reference handout, "Family Roles," to accompany the Handout # 40, "Family Roles Chart".

6. Provide the Family Roles and the Family Roles Chart Handout as the homework assignment for the follow-up group.

7. Ask the members to complete the identified roles in the Family Roles Chart, beginning with pre-school. The chart is only a guide to be used as the format. Ask the clients to change it as needed to explain divorces, deaths, siblings moving out, etc. If they did not marry, have them change their roles as jobs changed or include different relationships. As a variation, you can also keep the focus on their childhood years instead of including adult stages.

   Ask them to include their parents' roles. Usually, one parent is the codependent although this may change as children grow older and assume surrogate spouse roles.

Note: In the lecture provided, we have created one parent to be an addict. This may not be the case, and if not, the other parent assumes one of the identified roles. **For Example:** Mom is the Hero, Dad is the Lost Child, etc. **If there are more or less than three children, the roles become shared.** One child or parent could be both the Hero and Mascot, or Mascot and Scapegoat, or three children could be the Lost Child, etc.

Follow-Up Group: Distribute the "Family Roles Chart" Handout. Provide time to allow each client to diagram their Family Role Chart. When they are completed, ask them to diagram it on the blackboard. Help clarify their family roles and the effect it had on them. Ask the group to provide feedback.

Also include things such as:

Why did the roles change?
Which is your most comfortable role?
Which role do you revert back to under stress?
Who plays which roles in your current family/relationships?

For some groups, it may also be important to identify family strengths. This provides balance. It also empowers your clients to identify the strengths and gifts they developed to be able to recover. Ask your clients to identify three strengths they developed because of their family or in spite of their family (survivor skills), and how these strengths can affect their present.

HANDOUT #40

FAMILY ROLES CHART

Year	Mom	Dad	Child #1	Child #2	Child #3	How the role affected my past	How the role affects my present
Preschool							
Elem. School							
High School							
Before Marriage							
During Marriage							
Now							

ABUSE LECTURE

When our clients stopped drinking or using, they lost the primary tool they had to cope with stress, alcohol. They will no longer be able to instantly anesthetize themselves or transform underlying feelings of inadequacy, fear and shame. They will be walking into unknown territory — their feelings. For most chemical dependents, sobriety is a terrifying experience because they have not developed the ability to manage or handle their feelings, particularly their fear. This inability to soothe themselves and easily resolve conflict stems from childhood issues. An important piece of any treatment needs to include some examination of how those overwhelming and disturbing feelings from their childhood's exist in their psyches today and how they will affect their ability to stay sober.

To look at underlying fear and shame means accepting the need to explore and examine the childhood experiences from which their current dysfunctional emotional systems developed. To remove alcohol from our patients and ignore the issues related to their need for anesthesia is a form of therapeutic emotional neglect and abuse. Some addiction counselors explain to clients that their emotional pain is caused by their addiction, and that once the drinking stops, the pain will stop. This is simply false. Were it true, once detoxed, sobriety would be a snap. Why would anybody choose to drink again and create more pain?

The fact is, that for most drinkers, being chemically altered emotionally is far preferable to feeling real feelings. Hence the need to show your clients what it is they're trying to escape — a damaged sense of themselves and the inability to know how to heal these psychic wounds. How was this damaged sense of self created? In their childhoods, as a result of abuse.

This lecture is in four parts:

1. **Not recognizing abuse**
2. **The origins of abuse.**
3. **The development of abuse.**
4. **Recovery from abuse.**

Parts of the lecture are derived from the works of J. Konrad Stettbacher and Alice Miller.

PART I: NOT RECOGNIZING ABUSE

In their childhoods, our clients developed defense mechanisms for not perceiving abuse. Because of the nature of abuse being repetitive, children being limited in their cognitive responses, and a tremendous sense of disempowerment as a result of the abuse, the child is unable to recognize and confront the abuse. Therefore, to survive, the child develops defense mechanisms. **This is important, because as adults, these defenses will keep our clients from recognizing themselves as having been abused.** Their defense mechanisms are fully intact and operational. They have survived.

The first part of this lecture describes the defense mechanisms the client developed as a child that allowed their survival. Our clients don't recognize their abuse because they developed:

1. **Repression:** The absence of the memory. In this case, the abuse was so severe that it was simply blocked from memory. This is an unconscious process. The child cannot maintain the painful memory of the trauma and function from day to day, so the event and the memory is repressed.

Example: *"My sister says I was locked in a closet for two days. I can't remember it at all."*

2. **Suppression:** Consciously blocking a painful memory or event. Consciously choosing to forget the memory. The person can remember the event, but would rather block it.

Example: *"I can remember being locked in the closet, but I'd rather not think about it. I've gone years without thinking about it."*

3. **Dissociation:** A psychological separation of the persons' consciousness from their body when the abuse is perceived as being life threatening. The individual takes their "inner self" to safety where the abuse can't be felt, heard or seen. **Dissociation is the most severe form of defense and indicates perceived life threatening trauma.** The person disassociates to a place **outside** their body and in the most severe cases, into a black hole someplace **within** their body.

Example: *"I remember my father beating me. I can't remember the look on his face. How I remember it is as if I was standing over the incident, from the ceiling, looking down on it (or from the side)."*

The next three forms of defenses are less severe:

1. **Minimizing:** Decreasing the significance of the abuse to decrease the feelings around it, or its importance.

Example: *"I remember being hit. I didn't cry much. It wasn't a big deal."*

2. **Denial:** There's nothing wrong with the reality of the abuse.

Example: *"Sure I got hit. There's nothing wrong with that."*

3. **Delusion:** Believing something despite facts to the contrary. Seeing facts but not assigning proper meaning to them.

Example: *"Kids don't mind being hit. It doesn't hurt them. It's the only way to teach a child."*

List and review these defenses with your clients. Most of them will discover that while they use a variety of these defenses, they have a predominent mechanism. Which forms of defenses do they use? Which is their most effective defense?

PART II : ORIGINS OF ABUSE

This has been adapted from J. Konrad Stettbacker's book "Making Sense of Suffering."

In infancy, the child is totally dependent upon the caretaker to meet his or her needs. It is completely unable to obtain food or defend itself. The infant's survival is ultimately dependent upon the ability of the caretaker to meet his needs. For the child to develop trust, security, nurturing and growth, **all** of his needs must be consistently met. The way this looks in a **healthy child** is as follows:

Using the example of hunger :

1. The infant, Mary's, stomach is empty and Mary experiences her hunger as pain (the need).
2. Mary squeaks, (searching behavior).
3. Mother picks up Mary, holds her warmly and feeds her (object appraisal).
4. Mary experiences warm food and nurturing and becomes full. A pleasant experience.
5. Mary relaxes.
6. Mary rests.
7. Mary is hungry again, the cycle continues.

In its simplest form, the abuse cycle is set like this:

1. Mary is hungry, experiences a need.
2. Mary squeaks, searches for food.
3. Mother is tired, frustrated, distracted. She scowls at Mary while feeding her, or the milk is too hot. In any case, Mary can't know what the cause of her discomfort is — *she can not conceptualize Mother yet, she is far too young.* To feed and reduce the pain from the hunger, *she needs to be "blind" to Mother,* (object blindness.)
4. It is an uncomfortable experience (pain vs. pleasure).
5. Mary experiences tension (fear).
6. Mary can't relax.
7. Mary is hungry again. The cycle continues.

Because the infant is unable to identify the cause of their distress (Mother's anger or neglect, etc.), the child experiences pain. *If this cycle is repeated, the infant experiences* ***constant*** *dread and fear when she must have her needs met.* Due to her inability to perceive the reason that Mother is not able to meet Mary's needs (object blindness), Mary experiences fear of more pain when hungry. Mary can only experience herself. **Therefore, her hunger is to be feared.** Should this cycle be repeated, Mary will develop self-loathing and helplessness.

In infancy, the child is pre-cognizant. She has no words or theoretical framework. This cycle becomes apparent in her behavior of helplessness or rage. **She cannot meet her own needs.** Mother is "good," Mary and her feelings are "bad". **Over time this becomes sublimated, repressed, and transferred to objects as she becomes older.**

Now, as the child ages and develops verbally, **she has already developed defenses from her true feelings and reality.** Mary's sense of identity becomes lost in becoming attuned to Mother or Father's needs. Mother can't control her own anger or frustration, hits Mary, and tells Mary it's Mary's fault. Mary accepts this, and because of her repressed childhood, then transfers this pattern to her children because it was "good for Mary." **She is unable to recognize the abuse.**

Review the above section with your clients so they can understand the cycle.

PART III : THE DEVELOPMENT OF ABUSE

Review this with the group:

1. Abuse is about unequal power. The person with more power exerts their power over the person with less power.

2. Abuse exists in all areas of interactions: child to child, parent to child and vice versa, boss to employee, country to country.

3. The opposite of abuse is intimacy. *Intimacy is a relationship where there is equal power across the board.*

4. Abuse is generational. It passes from family to family. It is also cultural.

5. Abuse generates fear in the victim, or the person with less power. Fear of abandonment, fear of pain, fear of feeling shame, fear of more fear....

6. There are two types of abuse: **overt abuse** and **covert abuse. Overt abuse is obvious abuse.** It is also generational and cultural. In this Western culture, raping a three year old child is believed to be abusive. Overt abuse is abuse that is recognized as abuse within the culture.

   Covert abuse is "secret abuse." It is not abuse done in secret, rather it is **abuse done openly that states that it is not abuse. It is abusiveness that has been repressed.** For example, striking a child is abusive. Any form of **intentional damage to a child is abuse.** Children are totally defenseless. Because striking our children is acceptable in this culture, it is a form of covert abuse. The fact that it is a terrible form of abuse is kept secret with the delusion that "children need to be hit." When the Australian aborigines were told that Westerners struck their children as a matter of routine, the aborigines thought that the anthropologists had made it up. *They could not conceive nor comprehend the action of striking a child.* ***For any reason.***

In this next section, **on a blackboard,** go over the developmental sources of abuse. If the action caused fear, shame or some diminishing of the person, it is abuse.

Review the **ages** of developmental abuse and the **nature**, i.e., physical (includes sexual), emotional, and spiritual. Review whether the abuse was **covert** or **overt**. The structure looks like this:

		COVERT	**OVERT**
Age 0-2	**physical**		
	sexual		
	emotional		
	spiritual		
Age 2-6	**physical**		
	sexual		
	emotional		
	spiritual		
Age 6-12	**physical**		
	sexual		
	emotional		
	spiritual		
Age 13	**physical**		
(puberty)	**sexual**		
	emotional		
	spiritual		
Age 21	**physical**		
60	**sexual**		
82	**emotional**		
	spiritual		

(As a counselor, if you are not aware of the forms of abuse, review the materials by Alice Miller and other works about abuse or Adult Children of Alcoholics.)

Include in :

Physical abuse — hitting, slapping, pinching, tickling past the point of pleasure, not touching or nurturing.

Sexual abuse — poking, poor boundaries (nudity, open doors, inappropriate touching, shaming about sexuality, lying about the facts, sexual roles).

Emotional abuse — damaged ability to express all feelings, shaming, yelling, blaming, guilt.

Spiritual abuse — damaged creativity, sense of identity and purpose, wholeness. Also include the concept of "Who is God"? Is the parent God, or is "God" God?

Keep in mind that any behaviors that lead to shame are abusive.

This lecture could be given identically with the word "shame" substituted for abuse. A way to help your clients identify repressed shame is that shame is an intense feeling of being defective. Something is wrong with **me**.

An example to put on the blackboard to differentiate shame and guilt, is that

> Guilt is feeling bad about something **I've done**, out there.
> Shame is feeling bad about who **I am**, inside me.
> An example of a guilt statement is, "I can't believe I did **that**."
> An example of a shame statement is, "I can't believe **I** did that."

When your clients have completed the developmental sources of abuse, ask them to begin to identify what was common in their history. *At this stage, initial identification is the goal.* Their willingness to recount their personal histories are issues for group therapy.

The second part of the developmental sources of abuse requires some discussion about **how as children they coped with their abuse.** While they developed subconscious defenses as discussed initially, they **also** developed what some therapists call their "false self." The false self is essentially the parts of their personalities that **can cope** with both repressing the trauma while existing and functioning in their world.

This is an oversimplification but it works well with people in early recovery: The child experiences pain or fear or abandonment. To cope, they "seal off" those feelings and create another persona who can live in the world. The false self emerges, or a "mask" of another personality is put on and moves into the world.

For example:
Mary goes to the first grade. She is all excited — new friends, a shiny, new lunch box, her hair in curls, cute as can be. Within two hours, Mary experiences the abuse that is commonly allowed in first grade. She discovers that she is fat or skinny, her skin is the wrong color, curly hair is ugly, and her lunch box is uncool.
- If Mary was damaged as a child she will experience shame, fear, and isolation.
- If she experienced any form of abuse at home, she will not feel secure enough to tell her parents that she was abused in school and the true nature of her grief.
- **To cope, she will seal off her feelings and a false self will emerge which can cope with the torments.**

Some children have learned to adapt by developing aggressive false selves. These new emerging personalities will be aggressors — they will fight back, identify with their new abusers (object blindness), and become abusers themselves. Also, because they have repressed their pain, they won't be able to recognize it in others.

Other children will be passive. In sealing off their pain they will develop diffuse personalities to avoid notice. Still others will emerge as the class clown, the sports fanatic, etc.

Whichever defense can maintain repression and function in school will emerge as the false self or mask and become the dominant personality for as long as that "mask" is effective.

Should another abusive attack occur later in school, another false self will emerge to cope and repress the trauma and survive in the world. Frequent abusive situations include the onset of puberty, shaming over inability to grasp educational ideas, poor social skills, or their social "caste."

The creation of "false selves" is a similar dynamic as with the formation of family roles. The difference is that, unlike family roles where the role is assigned to the child **by the dysfunctional parent,** a false self emerges **from the child** **as a result of trauma.** Most of your clients will be able to recall the various "selves" they assumed and masks they wore throughout their childhood, adolescence and into the present.

In this exercise, ask your clients to recall the various personalities they developed. Once done, see if they can recall the **events** surrounding the experience and the **feelings** the new masks repressed.

This illustration demonstrates the concept to your clients. Draw it in stages on the blackboard as you describe each event.

Mary goes to first grade.

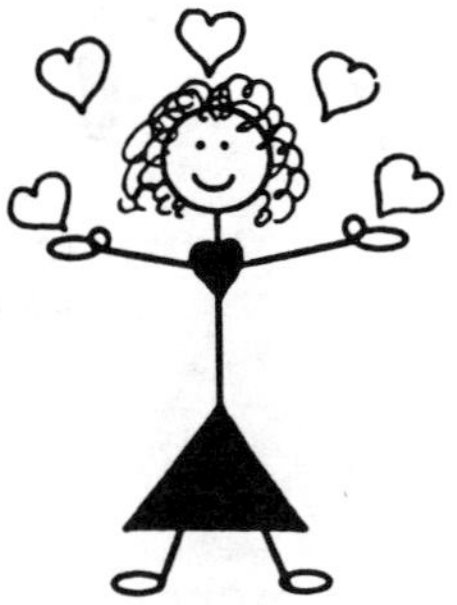

The event is racism and being called stupid.
The feelings are **shame**. She seals these feeling off and becomes **the perfect student.**

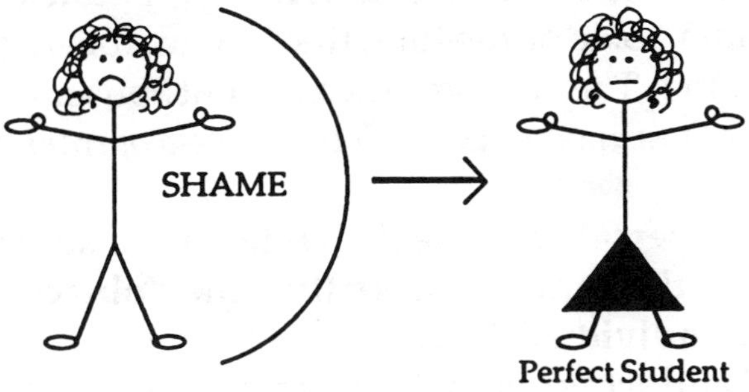

When she's ten-years-old, she gets picked on by older girls. She feels **afraid** and kicks them. They run away. Kicking people is a new way for her to not feel her fear or be picked on. She seals off her ability to feel fear and develops the **tough girl mask.**

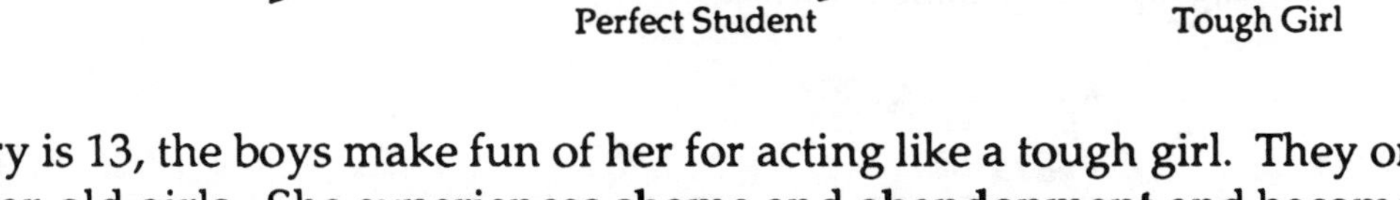

When Mary is 13, the boys make fun of her for acting like a tough girl. They only like the sexy 13-year-old girls. She experiences **shame** and **abandonment** and becomes a **"sexy" girl.**

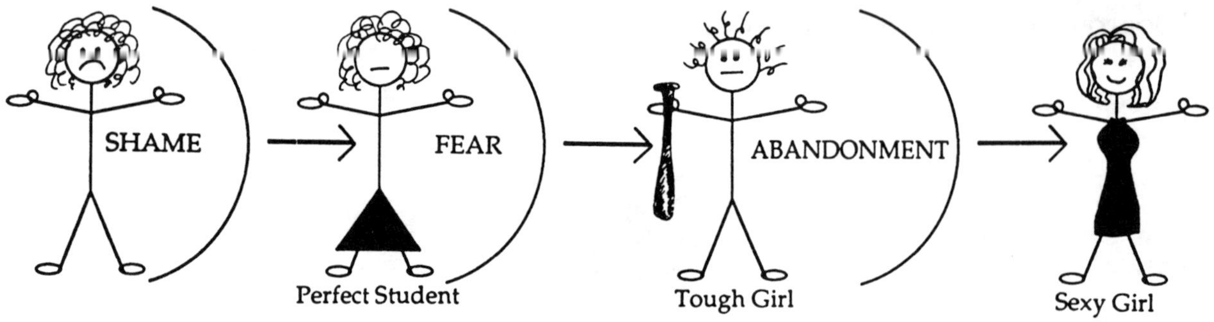

And so forth.

Layers upon layer of false selves emerge. Layers upon layer of feelings are repressed. This repression has numerous effects. First, the repressed feelings shown in the previous figures are intolerable to the individual. *Go back to the figures and circle those feelings for your client — shame, fear, abandonment.*

A person who can't feel shame behaves shamelessly. Because they are now unable to experience their own shame, toxic or healthy, they are unable to perceive it or empathize with others about their shame. They become inadvertent abusers. *This happens by repressing their shame and transferring it to another through the process of transference or projection.*

If shame is repressed, the person can't feel shame and is shameless. If the feeling is transferred or objectified, the individual loathes the "object" who now carries their shame. If, however, the individual is unable to repress or project their shame, they remain openly wounded and act as magnets, or caretakers, for others with this condition.

The same process happens with people who are not nurtured through their fear, abandonment issues, and grief. **Abused children become adults who have contempt for others and themselves, or repeat the behaviors by subconsciously becoming caretakers for others they perceive as experiencing abuse.** This is an oversimplification but your clients will understand the concepts.

Ask your clients to discuss how they coped with feelings of shame.

Has the shame been sealed off, projected or transferred to others?

Are they openly wounded caretakers with no boundaries?

It is very useful to have a separate follow-up group to spend more time with your clients simply discussing and detoxifying their shame issues.

PART IV : RECOVERY FROM ABUSE

Recovery from abuse occurs in stages and over time. Like recovery from alcoholism, it is important to stress that your clients can recover **if they are willing to go through all of the stages.** It is also imperative that the client work with a therapist or group who is willing to be their witness, their advocate, and stay with them through their journey.

STAGE 1 — In this initial stage, the client recalls the abuse. It involves eliciting memories as they are remembered, without regard for protecting the abusers. They simply remember what they had not been able or allowed to remember.

STAGE 2 — The client experiences the feelings and sensations they had previously blocked from their memory. They re-experience the repressed feelings and begin to identify how they were affected by the abuser.

STAGE 3 — The client questions and challenges the abuse. What was the explanation or justification for the abuse?

STAGE 4 — The client describes what they really need.

While this seems too short and too simple, **recovery is not more complicated than this.**

THE ABUSE TRIANGLE

This last section on abuse helps your clients identify how they are currently trapped in an abuse cycle. We would like to apologize for not recalling who first developed this cycle. It has been called the Victim Triangle and the Codependency Trap among others. For convenience sake and to fit with this lecture series, we will call it the Abuse Triangle.

Materials needed: Blackboard

Draw this triangle diagram on the board:

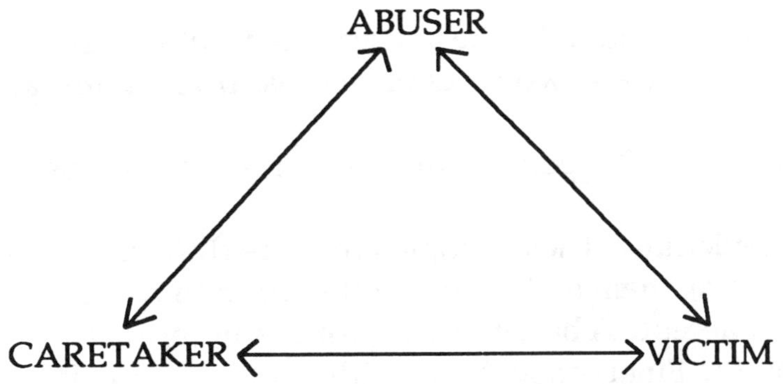

Depending upon the group, be they patients or families, different labels can be used in the triangle to identify the points around the triangle (**abuser** = perpetrator or addict; **caretaker** = codependent or rescuer; **victim** = survivor or scapegoat).

This cycle can work in three situations:

1. It can be the dynamic between three people.
2. It can be the dynamic between two people.
3. It can be the dynamic one person experiences.

All three will be explained.

When an individual has been raised or exposed to a dysfunctional family system, the Abuse Triangle dynamic occurs.

Definition of terms:

ABUSER — This person meets their needs by invading the boundaries of others. Their behavior is invasive and damaging to the integrity of another. These people are at some level out of control. Their out of control behavior provides relief to them, victimization to others.

Example #1 -- Intentional abuse or perpetration: A person who has lost control over their ability to create their own sense of power and rapes another. A person who strikes their child.

Example #2 -- "Unintentional" perpetration: A person who feels their own frustration and anger, can't integrate it within their structure and yells at another. Aggressive or passive-aggressive behavior is abusive.

VICTIM — This person is invaded by the abuser. They suffer some loss as a result of the perpetrator's behavior. There are two types of victims: **true victims** and **pseudo-victims.**

Example #1 -- True victims: The person walking home who is raped.

Example #2 -- Pseudo-victims: These people are more difficult to describe as they have complex dynamics keeping them in the victim role. To an "outsider", the victim role is not always simple to see or accept. A battered wife, for example, is clearly the victim of abuse when she shows up in the Emergency Room with a broken arm. When she refuses to go to a shelter or notify the police to apprehend her attacker, she becomes a pseudo-victim. The term pseudo-victim means that there is a secondary gain to remaining in the victim role. She may still love her husband, she may be afraid he will kill her if she calls the police, she may have no money or job skills, etc. Her secondary gains are security and so forth, *which are stronger than her ability to resolve and discard her victim role.*

Other types of pseudo-victims are those who meet their internal needs **by being victims.** Again, the dynamic is a complex one. For whatever reasons, these people are most "comfortable" being victims. "Martyrs" are an example of this. Their internal needs are met **through others responding to their victimization.** The woman who refuses to go to Al-Anon yet calls her friends daily eliciting sympathy by describing her drinking husband's abuse is an example of this. She meets her needs through this form of control, remaining a victim.

CARETAKERS — These people meet their internal needs through rescuing, enabling, and controlling others. They are usually responding to internal fear and abandonment issues and find relief from these feelings by being indispensable to others. Fixing them. Caretakers interact with the victims: *"Your father didn't mean to hit you"* and they interact with the abusers: *"I know you didn't mean to hurt her"*. **Caretakers never confront reality as this would jeopardize their position and elicit their unconscious abandonment issues.**

THE THREE PERSON ABUSE TRIANGLE:

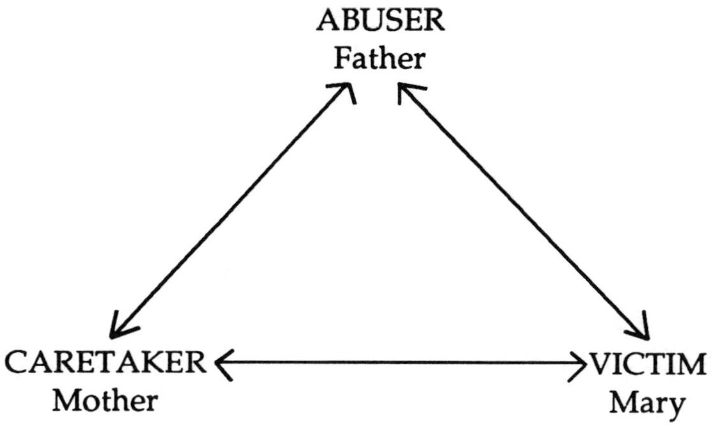

This is a stereotypical example but it is easiest to explain:

Father is the alcoholic and therefore the **Abuser.** The fact is that alcoholism and alcoholics abuse others.
Mother is the **Caretaker.**
Daughter, Mary, is the **Victim.**

Father is drunk and screams at Mary. His behavior is **abusive** and he creates the **victim,** Mary.
Mother is the **caretaker** for Father, "I know you didn't mean to yell at her," and to Mary, "he really loves you."

The following morning, Father apologizes to Mary.
Mary screams, "Go F— yourself! I wish you were dead!"
Father sulks off.
Mother rushes off to comfort poor Father and to calm down Mary.
Now Mary is the abuser, Father is the victim. Mother fixes them both.

Mary confronts Mother on her enabling Father's alcoholism and his behavior last night.
Mother tells Mary to mind her own business, that Father is not an alcoholic.
Because she is dishonest, Mother becomes the abuser, Mary the victim. Actually, Mary is a double victim. She is a victim to Mother's dishonesty, and Mother also fails to protect her child from an abusive alcoholic parent.

In the three person cycle, **the positions are interchangeable,** with all three people capable of rotating positions. Usually, however, each person is most comfortable within a primary role and will replay the dynamic until they are back in their comfort zone and "homeostasis" is maintained. Mother will end her day as the Caretaker, Mary the Victim, and Father will always be the Abuser if he's drinking.

THE TWO PERSON ABUSE TRIANGLE:

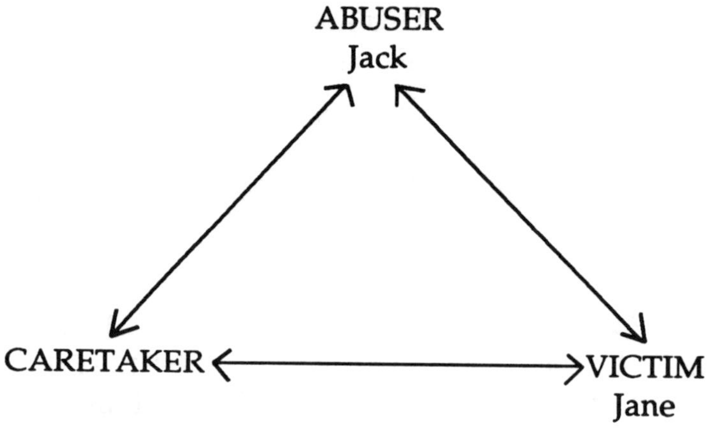

In this scenario, all three positions are played by two people. Jack comes home drunk and screams at Jane. Jack is the **abuser**, Jane the **victim**. Jack sobers up, feels bad and brings home flowers. He becomes the **caretaker**. Jane yells at him, becoming the **abuser**. Jane regrets yelling, makes his favorite dinner, and becomes the **caretaker**. The cycle goes around.

THE ONE PERSON ABUSE TRIANGLE:

I yell at my employees. **I am abusive.** I have hurt their feelings. I bring them donuts to make up for my behavior. **I am caretaking.** They ignore me. **I feel like the victim,** poor me.

or

My friend asks me to lend him rent money. I do. **I am caretaking.** He doesn't pay me back within a month. I need the money for my car payment. **I am the victim.** I talk about him behind his back, **I am abusive.**

I can play all three roles by myself.

Rule #1 about the Triangle (There's only one) :

Once a person **engages** in behaviors in the triangle, they are compelled to continue the cycle.

Once in the cycle, there is no way out of the roles!!

To quit the abuse triangle, there is a very simple solution.

DON'T ENTER THE CYCLE !!

This is the only solution.

Don't be a caretaker.
Don't be an abuser.
Don't be a victim.
If you are doing it, stop.

Easier said than done, right? Right! This is a wonderful juncture to reinforce to family members the need for continued therapeutic support. It's much easier to stop destructive behaviors with help.

Remind the group that if they choose to change their behaviors, and **not** engage in the Abuse Triangle anymore, the others who were in the dynamic will still try to keep them in their old roles. **Unless the family gets into recovery, the family will still play out the roles.** This is frequently seen when the alcoholic gets into recovery but their significant other does not.

For example, using the two person cycle: The addict, Jack, stops using, caretaking and being a victim. Jane won't go to Al-Anon, she doesn't have a problem. If Jack spends time in AA, Jane feels left out. She is a "victim" and perceives Jack as leaving her for his "new friends." So Jane maintains her victim role by saying that Jack is still abusive to her. **This behavior of hers is actually abusive.** Jane continues around the Triangle without Jack.

In the one person cycle, if the person changes only one behavior, they will always have the remaining two pathologies to contend with.

Follow Up Group:

Ask your clients to identify how they engage in all three cycles using specific examples. Ask them to identify new behaviors. This is best given as a homework assignment with the individual presenting their cycle to the group and receiving feedback. Be certain to ask for specific new healthy behaviors. The assertiveness and boundary exercises will help them concretize their specific healthy behaviors.

NOTES TO THE CLINICIAN :

The most difficult role to address in the Abuse Triangle is the person who stays in the victim role. There seems to be two reasons for this. First, the victim is usually initially a true victim, or survivor of childhood abuse. Their childhood helplessness and defenselessness become ingrained in their personality structure and coping skills. An example of this is found in the borderline or passive/passive-dependent personalities. They constantly "split off" from, or are unable to access, a core personality that can take responsibility and set limits and boundaries. This happened as the result of childhood abuse and trauma. Usually, two requirements are necessary to assist these people to move out of their victim role -- childhood abuse therapy (see Abuse Lecture), in combination with behavioral modification, as in scaling questions and chair work that focuses on ego strengths.

The second reason these people are difficult to help is that when their fragile victim roles are "threatened," **they attack.** Nearly 100% of victims become abusers. Their abuse is very subtle, but highly toxic. **As they have poor ego identification, their identities are attached to being victims. To be able to cope, they need to remain victims.** To remain victims means that they need an abuser. Anybody will do. Preferably the person who usually abuses them, but if that person disengages, the victim will transfer and project their feelings onto the next available source (like their counselor).

The way this is portrayed in a relationship is as follows:

- Jane has always been the victim of Jack's abusive drinking and behavior.
- Jack quits drinking, goes to AA and gets therapy. Within six months, Jack has learned to identify his feelings, be assertive and he is more peaceful.
- Jane says, "Why are you still so mean to me?"
- **Jack has not been mean at all.** In fact, Jack is more kind to Jane than ever. He explains this to Jane.
- Jane says, "Now you are yelling at me."

Jane's subconscious need to be a victim is highly abusive. Her abusiveness toward Jack is subtle but highly damaging. This can and usually goes further. Jane continues to tell her friends that Jack is still mean to her (more abuse to Jack). She cries all day long and accuses Jack of not loving her anymore (which he does), etc.

Untreated victims are highly abusive. The way that the victim becomes abusive needs to be explained to your group. Most of them are in these relationship triangles. They will not be able to recognize the perpetrative behaviors their "victims" are now inflicting upon them.

This is an excellent presentation for a mixed group of addicts and their families. If your clients have relationship conflicts, **constantly** ask them to identify how the roles have shifted in this dynamic so that they may become more adept at recognizing the problems and the solutions.

MULTIPLE FAMILY GROUP

This is a group designed for treatment participants, family, and friends who are part of the Family Education Program. We have developed the format to last 1 1/2 hours, once a week for four weeks.

Objective: To provide a structured safe environment which promotes direct communication between family members about the impact of alcoholism and codependency on their relationships.

In the Family Education Program, the core groups preparing them for this work include:

Codependency
Disease Concepts
The Developmental Process of Recovery

Materials needed: Blackboard.

Setting up the room: Arrange chairs in a circle. Place two chairs in the center of the circle. Place tissue within reach of the center chairs.

1. **Introductions.**

2. **Confidentiality statement:** "Who you see her, what you hear here, let it stay here. It is important that all of us make this a safe place to speak freely."

3. **Directions to the group:** Each family will come to the center of the circle, beginning with the family who has been in treatment the longest. When speaking and listening to each, other it is important to be direct. This might feel a little awkward at first. **Guidelines that will help:**

   - Look directly at the person you are addressing.
   - Speak directly to the person saying "you" (rather than "him" or "my mother").
   - Assume a body posture of openness by avoiding crossing your arms or crossing your legs. (The therapist should demonstrate open body posture.)

Each person in the center chairs will use the statement which applies to themselves (written on the board) and complete the statements **as they relate to themselves.** The counselors may stop the client to help them stay with the subject or to be more direct with each other.

The family members may not respond until each person has completed the exercise. The group interacts with the family in the center by giving them feedback and support. Advice giving is not allowed at any time.

If a client has no family attending, he will chose someone from the group to represent a significant family member to complete their part of the exercise. The person filling in **does not** respond to the codependent's part in the exercise.

Note: These topics and statements are written on the board before the group begins. We strongly recommend two therapist to co-facilitate.

Week I: The Effects of the Disease

Treatment Participant: "One way that my alcoholism/ addiction has affected my relationship with you is__________. In my recovery, I commit to__________. Another way my alcoholism affected my relationship with you is____________. In my recovery, I commit to_______."

Codependent: "One way that your alcoholism has affected me is________. In my recovery, I commit to__________. Another way your alcoholism/addiction has affected me is___________. In my recovery, I commit to___________."

Week II: Blame and Responsibility

Treatment Participant: "One way that I have blamed you for my using is_________. The truth is________. From now on I am responsible for_______. Another way that I have blamed you for my using is______. The truth is_________. From now on I am responsible for_________."

Codependent: "One way that I have blamed something or someone else for your using is_______. The truth is________. From now on I am responsible for________. Another way that I have blamed something or someone else for your using is __________. The truth is_______. From now on I am responsible for________."

Week III: Enabling (Give definition of enabling)

Treatment Participant: "One way that you have enabled me is_______. The truth is ______. I commit to_______.
Another way that you have enabled me is________. The truth is________. I commit to______."

Codependent: One way that I have enabled you is_______. The truth is_______. I commit to_______.
Another way I have enabled you is_______. The truth is_________. I commit to_________."

Week IV: Openness

All Participants: "One thing I need to talk to you about is_______. When I talk to you about this I expect to feel_________. I commit to talk to you about this (set a time)_______."

Alternative topic: Lies

Treatment Participant: "One lie that I told to you about my using was_______. The truth is________. From now on I commit to______.
Another lie that I told you was______. The truth is________. From now on I commit to________."

Codependent: "One lie that I told to someone else about your using was______. The truth is_______. From now on I commit to______.
Another lie I told to someone is_______. The truth is______. From now on I commit to________."

Notes To Clinicians :
This group will require a lot of redirection. Members often have their own agenda. To maintain the integrity of the group, remind the members that you will redirect them as needed to stay on track.

Also, directing participants to remain in an open body posture is important throughout. Suggest when speaking and listening that each person sit with their hands flat on their laps or upper legs. The tendency will be a defensive stance with arms folded across the chest. Stop the interaction when necessary to ask the person to resume an open position. **Tell participants ahead of time that you will be interrupting if they need help in being direct with addressing each other.**

When the exercise has been completed by all participants, allow time for the group to process what it was like to share and listen to each other.

RELAPSE

Notes To Clinicians:

Relapse plays an important role in all our treatment programs. We need to consider our own expectations and definitions of relapse and recovery. If we review statistics on relapse, we find that they are not reliable. Studies related to relapse are difficult and tend to be inaccurate.

We do know that the majority of alcoholics relapse during their first year of sobriety. Relapse is a common symptom of chemical dependency. We have also begun to see a trend toward rising relapse rates for clients in treatment.

There are several significant influences which are changing the profile of the chemically dependent person in treatment settings. Treatment is promoted to a much higher degree as evidenced by increasing numbers of referrals to treatment by the courts and by employers. The influence of Managed Health Care also has a dramatic impact on the quality of treatment available. The trend toward briefer and more cost effective treatment challenges us to prioritize. Many of us are redesigning programming and schedules to meet these new demands.

We have personally seen an increase in relapse for clients in the out-patient setting and a small percentage of clients who have not achieved any abstinence at all. Clearly the challenge of dealing with relapse in treatment is growing. The fact is that abstinence may not necessarily be the measure of success in treatment. Is it possible for a client to drink in treatment **and still find recovery?** Due to these new constraints and our decreased ability to provide adequate services, it is important for facilities to define relapse and have a clear strategy for working with it.

Working with clients to use relapse as a part of their recovery experience can be useful. It can reinforce the understanding of "powerlessness" over the disease, turning failure into an opportunity to enhance recovery. For some, it can make the "first step" of sobriety come alive and strengthen commitment to recovery.

As clinicians, we all have a responsibility individually and as part of the treatment team to review and consider how we define relapse and recovery, and to clarify treatment expectations.

THE DEVELOPMENTAL PROCESS OF RECOVERY

This group works well for a combined audience of chemically dependent clients and their codependent supports. It is presented in a lecture with intermittent group participation. The material is important in preparing clients and families for the milestones they will face in recovery. The lecture format contains the basic points and is designed to be a guide in presentation.

Materials needed: Blackboard, Handouts # 41, 42, 43, and 44.

> Place "The Developmental Process Of Recovery" graph on the blackboard prior to the group, labeling the stages of recovery. (See Handout # 41.)

Recovery is a developmental process. In each stage we complete specific tasks and learn something new which prepares us for the next stage.

1. **The "honeymoon" or "pink cloud" stage:**

   This phase begins after completion of detox. The client is feeling better. Ask the group what some of the benefits are for them in this stage and *list them on the board.* **For example:** Feeling better physically, or relief for the codependent. *There is a tendency for addicts and significant others to attach unrealistic expectations to sobriety.* Not everyone experiences a "pink cloud." Some may face consequences of their disease, such as loss of their job or relationships. **The task during the "Pink Cloud" phase is to be realistic about the problems that exist for them.**

   Example: *"All of our problems were related to using, therefore, everything will run smoothly now!"*

2. **Reality Stage (Five to Seven Weeks):**

   At this stage, reality sets in. What are some of the problems which continue after sobriety? What are some new problems associated with sobriety? *Generate a list of group responses.* **Example:** financial problems, making changes in social life. **The task of this phase is to solve problems and manage difficulties without using.**

   There is a significant rate of relapse at this stage. As we move through this phase we gain some solid recovery experience. We have learned new ways to address old problems. We begin to revive interests, goals and activities lost in our using. We are working a recovery program and it is working for us.

3. Decisions (Six Months):

At this point, a lot of clients feel they should make a major life change. Considering the circumstances, what kind of decisions or changes do you envision in your life? *List group responses.* **Example:** Marriage, divorce, buying a house. The problem with making major life changes is that significant life change is accompanied by stress. Stress occurs whether the change has positive or negative consequences. The more drastic the change, the greater the stress.

The suggestion in recovery is to "avoid making major decisions in the first year of sobriety." *Explore reasons for this suggestions with the group.* **The task of this phase is to create a balanced life style and to begin to repair the "wreckage of the past."** An increase in stress often results in relapse of other compulsive behaviors, such as over-working or over-eating.

4. I Can Do It Myself (One Year):

The desire to use is greatly curtailed and a sense of control over the disease is experienced at this stage. What might you expect to see at this stage? *List group responses on the board.* Behaviors include reducing or discontinuing participation in AA/NA. This, too, is a time of significant relapse. **The task at this point is to re-engage in a recovery program, increasing meetings and reworking the Twelve Steps with a sponsor.**

5. Emotional Recovery:

In the late recovery stage, beginning at about 18 months of sobriety, underlying emotional issues begin to surface. These issues are related to our childhood and family dynamics. They affect our behavior and relations with others. This is the time to begin therapy. **The task is to continue growth towards emotional health and the achievement of intimacy with those we love.** Some may benefit from therapy earlier in sobriety. Pay attention to your emotional condition.

The key to success in the recovery process is working a recovery program.

See Handout #43, Recovery Suggestions. *Review these briefly with the group.*

Relapse:

Here are a few points to reinforce, related to relapse:

1. **"Relapse happens before it happens".** Relapse is a process of returning to using chemicals after a period of abstinence. Picking up the drink or drug is the last act of the process. Denial kept us using and that same denial will bring us back.

2. **"If I do what I did, I get what I got."** In order to stay sober, behavior must change.

   Regular review of the handout "Warning Signs Of Relapse" can assist in identifying thoughts and behaviors which can lead to relapse.

3. **Relapse statistics are not reliable.** We know that more than two-thirds of addicts relapse in the first year of sobriety. We also know that alcoholics and addicts who receive treatment and work a recovery program have a better chance of maintaining sobriety than those who do not go into treatment.

HANDOUT #41

DEVELOPMENTAL PROCESS OF RECOVERY

Pink Cloud or Honeymoon	Reality	Decisions	I can do it myself	Emotional Recovery

Feelings

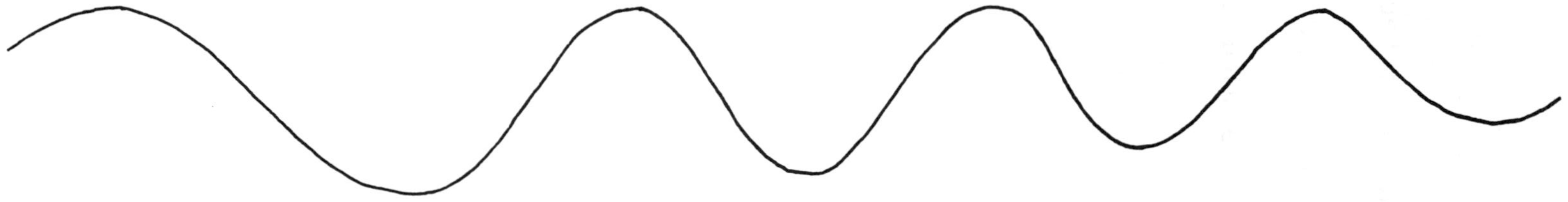

Pink Cloud or Honeymoon	Reality	Decisions	I can do it myself	Emotional Recovery
	5 - 7 weeks	6 months	12 months	18 months
"I feel great" Court worked out Relationships OK Job is OK	"I hate my job" Kids are angry Spouse not working a program Too many responsibilities No friends Mood swings Bored Lonely Less socializing as a couple Spouse is irritable/ controlling Still fighting over same old things Alcoholic is out too much at meetings Unrealistic expectations	Divorce Marriage Have a baby Change jobs Move Buy a house Go back to school Buy a car	"I don't need meetings." "I don't need a sponsor:" Stop working the steps Codependents drop out of Al-Anon— "All fixed"	Emotional issues Surface Relationships Family issues Childhood issues Time for counseling
Task: Be realistic about existing problems	**Task: Solve problems and manage difficulties without using**	**Task: Work toward lifestyle balance and repairing the wreckage of the past**	**Task: Recommit to recovery program**	**Task: Continue growth toward emotional health and achievement of intimacy in relationships**

* NOTE: Emotional highs and lows are more severe in early recovery. The feelings graph shows that as each stage is resolved, we feel better and mood swings become less severe and less frequent.

HANDOUT #42

STRESS LIST

These events are listed in order of severity of stress. Note those that currently apply to you. Remember that all change creates stress. An important part of recovery is learning healthy ways to cope with it and using discretion when planning major life changes.

EVENT:

Death of a child or spouse.
Death of a family member.
Physical injury or major illness.
Marriage.
Being fired from a job.
Marital reconciliation.
Physical illness of family member.
Pregnancy.
Sexual problems.
New baby or adoption.
Financial changes.
Death of a close friend.
Changing careers.
Increases in arguments with significant others.
Mortgage payments.
Foreclosure, Bankruptcy.
Increased expectations at work.
Children leaving home.
Outstanding personal achievement.
Partner loses or starts job.
Going back to school.
Graduating from school.
Change in living condition.
Change in personal habits.
Difficulties with boss.
Change in work schedule.
Change in residence.
Change in church activities.
Change in social activities.
Change in sleep pattern.
Increase or decrease in family contact.
Change in eating habits.
Vacation.
Christmas.
Minor law violations.

HANDOUT #43

RECOVERY SUGGESTIONS

Meetings: In AA, it is recommended that those starting out in recovery attend 90 meetings in 90 days. For Al-Anon, we recommend a minimum of two meetings per week.

Sponsor: Find a sponsor. A sponsor is somebody in the "program" who has already gone through recovery stages. They can support and guide you in your recovery process.

The 12 Steps: Work the Steps. The 12 Steps provide an emotional and spiritual framework for recovery.

Service: Active involvement in AA or Al-Anon.

Prayer And Meditation: Finding a way for spiritual expression that works for us is an individual decision. Allowing each other this freedom is absolutely necessary in recovery.

Literature: This refers to reading *The Big Book, Twelve and Twelve,* and Al-Anon literature.

Home Group: Joining a group and committing to regular attendance at that meeting helps us engage with others in the program and become "a part of."

The good news is that following these suggestions practically ensures successful recovery. The bad news is that most of us are terrible at following suggestions.

The choice is yours!

HANDOUT #44

RELAPSE WARNING SIGNS

_____ Trying to control or run another's recovery program

_____ Isolating

_____ Depression

_____ Compulsive or impulsive behaviors

_____ Attempts to control people, places, and things

_____ Being defensive

_____ I don't care attitude

_____ Taking on the responsibilities of others

_____ Anger easily

_____ Day dreaming

_____ Lying

_____ Holding feelings in

_____ Periods of confusion

_____ Feeling powerless and hopeless

_____ Feeling sorry for myself

_____ Preoccupation with one area of my life

_____ Over-reaction to stressful situations

_____ Over or under sleeping

_____ Over or under eating

_____ Loss of daily structure

_____ Feelings of inferiority or superiority

_____ Nagging/whining

_____ Immature wish to be happy or make others happy

_____ Insensitivity to the feelings of others

_____ Avoiding dealing with issues or problems

_____ Try to force sobriety on others

_____ Focusing on the past

_____ Projecting into the future

_____ Not having any fun

_____ Compulsive sexual behavior

_____ Hoarding money or over-spending

_____ Increasing physical complaints

_____ Fantasies about social drinking

_____ Increasing work dissatisfaction

_____ Over-confidence about recovery

_____ Increasing use of non prescription medication

_____ Rejecting help

_____ Blaming others for my problems

_____ Cutting down or stopping meetings

_____ Resentments

_____ Hanging around using environments

_____ Thinking I am cured

_____ Start using a chemical other than my drug of choice

_____ Convince myself I can practice controlled drinking

_____ Lose control

_____ Deny my fears

_____ See problems as unsolvable

_____ Unrealistic expectations

WHAT TO DO:

Go to a meeting
Call your sponsor
Talk about it — ask for help
Read program literature
Make a daily inventory

RELAPSE HAPPENS BEFORE IT HAPPENS

Objectives:

1. The client will understand the concept of relapse as a process.

2. The client will identify his own external and internal warning signs of relapse.

3. The client will identify tools and behavior which can interrupt the relapse process.

Materials needed: Blackboard, Relapse Warning Sign List, Pencils

Opening Discussion:

Relapse happens before it happens. "Relapse is a process, not an event". The relapse process reactivates the symptoms of our disease, ultimately bringing us back to using/ drinking. If all it took to recover was to see and admit to having the disease, then relapse would not be a problem. Unfortunately, the disease of alcoholism is more complicated than that. We have denial which doesn't leave us overnight. To uncover denial requires that we be honest, open, and willing. Willing to admit our faulty thinking and see the real truth.

In recovery, **we cannot make denial go away.** It is a symptom and it is here to stay. We can uncover it on a daily basis, however, and address it in our program. If we do not notice our denial, it will go back underground. Relapse at this point is probably inevitable. Our recovery is dependent on our ability to recognize and manage denial on a daily basis.

Identifying the warning signs of relapse will show us our denial. Doing something about the warning signs will help us to recover. For example: As alcoholics/addicts, we have learned to lie as a means of protection for our using, feelings, thinking, and behavior. When we stop using, we may stop lying about it, but we will continue to lie about the rest. An addict at any point of recovery, if he has maintained awareness of his denial, will notice when he lies. The reasons for lying are always the same. *"I don't want you to know what I really feel, think, or do."* Recovery does not assume that we will stop lying, but rather teaches us to go back and tell the truth after we have lied. When we practice this enough, we will find that we lie less. **It's progress not perfection.**

Taking a daily inventory of feelings, thinking, and behavior will help us recognize our denial and give us the opportunity to do something about it.

1. Distribute the Handout # 44, "Relapse Warning Signs". Ask the group to make a decision to be honest, open, and willing as they review the list in the Handout. They may only check off the signs apply to them, today and for which they can give a specific example.

   Take ten minutes to complete the assignment.

2. Ask the group to break into pairs. If you have an odd number there will be one group with three members. Ask one person in the pair to begin by sharing a warning sign that applies to them and his example. Have the pair rotate back and forth. Allow twenty minutes for the exchange.

3. Re-group: Have a brief discussion period. What was it like to do the exercise? Was it difficult to find warning signs that applied to you? What was it like telling someone else?

4. On the blackboard, make two columns labeled Relapse Warning Sign and Recovery Action. Ask each client individually to share one example and one warning sign with the group. Write in on the board. Ask the client what action can he/she take today to address it.

Example:

NAME:	**RELAPSE WARNING SIGN:**	**RECOVERY ACTION:**
Mary:	Hanging around using environment.	Talk about it in AA tonight. Talk to my sponsor about missing my using friends.
Brad:	Stopped by bar last night.	Make plans to go to a movie with a sober friend in treatment.

Ask the group if they have any other ideas for Mary to add to the action list.
Ask Mary what commitment she can make to address this warning sign **today.**
Example: *"I will talk about going to the bar in the meeting tonight."*
Write down each individual's commitment.
Follow-Up the next day to allow clients to let the group know if in fact they did follow-through, and if not, discuss what prevented them from taking the action.

HANDOUT #44

RELAPSE WARNING SIGNS

_____ Trying to control or run another's recovery program

_____ Isolating

_____ Depression

_____ Compulsive or impulsive behaviors

_____ Attempts to control people, places, and things

_____ Being defensive

_____ I don't care attitude

_____ Taking on the responsibilities of others

_____ Anger easily

_____ Day dreaming

_____ Lying

_____ Holding feelings in

_____ Periods of confusion

_____ Feeling powerless and hopeless

_____ Feeling sorry for myself

_____ Preoccupation with one area of my life

_____ Over-reaction to stressful situations

_____ Over or under sleeping

_____ Over or under eating

_____ Loss of daily structure

_____ Feelings of inferiority or superiority

_____ Nagging/whining

_____ Immature wish to be happy or make others happy

_____ Insensitivity to the feelings of others

_____ Avoiding dealing with issues or problems

_____ Try to force sobriety on others

_____ Focusing on the past

_____ Projecting into the future

_____ Not having any fun

_____ Compulsive sexual behavior

_____ Hoarding money or over-spending

_____ Increasing physical complaints

_____ Fantasies about social drinking

_____ Increasing work dissatisfaction

- _____ Over-confidence about recovery
- _____ Increasing use of non prescription medication
- _____ Rejecting help
- _____ Blaming others for my problems
- _____ Cutting down or stopping meetings
- _____ Resentments
- _____ Hanging around using environments
- _____ Thinking I am cured
- _____ Start using a chemical other than my drug of choice
- _____ Convince myself I can practice controlled drinking
- _____ Lose control
- _____ Deny my fears
- _____ See problems as unsolvable
- _____ Unrealistic expectations

WHAT TO DO:

Go to a meeting
Call your sponsor
Talk about it — ask for help
Read program literature
Make a daily inventory

RELAPSE PREVENTION PLAN

(Note - this group is Handout # 45.)
Relapse is common for alcoholics and addicts. We do not have to relapse. Preventing relapse requires an awareness of our own denial process and the willingness to do something about it. We need to be vigilant about exposing our denial to ourselves and others.

I. You have the information within yourself that tells you the circumstances which can set you up for relapse. Answer the following questions as honestly as you can.

Who are the people you are most likely to use with?

1.

2.

3.

4.

5.

What feelings place you at greatest risk for using?

1.

2.

3.

What situations or events place you at risk for using? Why?

1.

2.

3.

4.

5.

What will be the consequences for you if you relapse?

1.

2.

3.

4.

II. This plan is used in conjunction with your Relapse Warning List. You may use this list as part of a daily inventory to check on your denial status, and plan your recovery day around it. Review the list. Identify your warning signs. Look at your feelings, thoughts, behavior, and decide what you will do about it.

Example:

Warning sign: Hanging around using environments.

Thought/s: I miss my friends.

Feeling/s: I feel bored and lonely.

Behavior: I stopped at the bar just to say hello. I had a coke.

Recovery Action:
a. Call my sponsor and talk to him/her about it.
b. Go to a meeting and talk about it.
c. Make plans to go to a movie with a sober friend in treatment.

Warning Sign:

Thought/s:

Feeling/s:

Behavior:

Recovery Action:
a.
b.
c.

Warning Sign:

Thought/s:

Feeling/s:

Behavior:

Recovery Action: a.
b.
c.

Warning Sign:

Thought/s:

Feeling/s:

Behavior:

Recovery Action: a.
b.
c.

Warning Sign:

Thought/s:

Feeling/s:

Behavior:

Recovery Action: a.
b.
c.

Warning Sign:

Thought/s:

Feeling/s:

Behavior:

Recovery Action: a.
b.
c.

RECOVERY PLAN AND RECOVERY PLAN OUTLINE :

Notes To Clinicians :

This last section deals with the client's recovery, or aftercare plan. You have been provided with two parts:

The "Recovery Plan Outline", Handout #46, uses examples to demonstrate the content and structure of a comprehensive Recovery Plan. We suggest reviewing it as a Handout in the group setting. This gives all of the clients the benefit of hearing each other's and your responses.

- The "Recovery Plan", Handout #47, is the plan itself.
- The client is to complete the plan and review it with their counselor.
- Only after being reviewed should it be signed by the client and staff.
- Remind the client to write it in pen as the plan will go into their chart as their exit note or discharge plan.
- Provide the client with a copy (not the original) for their personal use and/or to give to the Aftercare Co-ordinator upon discharge.

RECOVERY PLAN OUTLINE

The recovery plan is a 90-day contract that we make with ourselves specifically detailing the action that we will take in our own recovery. **This is a commitment** and to ensure success, it needs to be realistic. KEEP IT SIMPLE!

A commitment is a **decision**. The best way to express a commitment is to firmly state what our action will be. The words "I will" show a decision to follow through with action. For example, please note the difference in the following two statements:

> **1.** "I will go to an AA meeting every day for 90 days."
>
> **2.** "I will try to go to an AA meeting every day."

In AA they say, *"Trying is Lying"* or *"Trying is Dying"*. Trying means that there is really no commitment at all! We can always let ourselves off the hook with *"Oh well, I tried."* Our commitment should be **simple, clear,** and **realistic**. For instance, if I am considering some form of exercise in my sober program and I have been a "couch potato" for the last five years, then a commitment to run ten miles a day is unreasonable. Instead, I could commit to walking to work and back every day. It would be a ten minute walk each way and my commitment would be: *"I will walk a total of twenty minutes five days per week."* The statement includes **what I will do** and **how often I will do it.**

The following outline may help to design your own individual recovery plan:

ALWAYS INCLUDE <u>WHAT</u> AND <u>HOW OFTEN</u> !!!!

1. Remaining chemically free: What chemicals will enter your body?

Example:

"I will remain chemically free, one day at a time. I will inform my physician that I am a recovering alcoholic. I will inform my dentist that I am a recovering alcoholic. I will check out all medications I may need with my sponsor or the treatment program."

2. **Meetings:** When, where, and how often will you go to meetings?

Examples:

"I will attend 90 meetings in 90 days." If you already know that you can't attend a meeting on a certain day, "double up" the following day. Include a tentative meeting schedule:

Example:

"I will attend 90 meetings in 90 days. Every other Monday I have class so I can't make a meeting. Therefore I will double-up meetings on Tuesday by attending the noon and 6 PM meetings."

3. **Sponsorship:** Who is my sponsor? How often will I contact him/her? If I do not have a sponsor, will I get one? When will I get one?

Examples:

1. My sponsor's name is Ann. I will call her every other day.

2. I will have a sponsor in one week.

3. I am moving to Santa Fe when I leave treatment. I will have a temporary sponsor within two weeks of my arrival.

4. **Working The Steps:**

Examples:

1. I will review my Step One with my sponsor next week.

2. I will continue working the Steps and meet with my sponsor every two weeks.

(Remember, you cannot complete this one unless you have consulted with your sponsor.)

5. **Spirituality:** How do you get in touch with your spiritual self and have time for contemplation? Include a plan for prayer and meditation, religious practices if appropriate.

   Examples:

   1. I will read my Twenty-Four Hour Book every morning.
   2. I will pray every morning and every evening.
   3. I will attend church services every two weeks with my family.
   4. I will take a walk in the woods once a week.

6. **Physical Health:** Include commitment for diet, exercise, medical problems.

   Examples:

   1. I will continue treatment for my gastric ulcer and will follow-up with my physician. I have an appointment on ____________.
   2. I will eat at least two healthy meals per day.
   3. I will work out at the gym two times per week.
   4. I will take my high blood pressure medication as prescribed by my physician.

7. **Emotional Health:** Include any counseling appointments and the name of the counselor or who you will talk with about your feelings.

   Examples:

   1. I will talk to my sponsor at least two times per week about my feelings.
   2. I will share my feelings with my husband as they come up instead of holding them in.
   3. I will follow through with my counseling appointment with __________ on __________.

Identify the feeling that is most difficult for you to deal with.

Example: Anger.

When you are angry, what will you do to deal with it?

1. Go to a meeting and talk about it.
2. Call my sponsor or a sober friend.
3. When I have a fight with my wife, I will go for a ten minute walk to calm down.

8. **Employment:** What are your work plans? Since overworking is often a compulsive behavior and can interfere with your program, what is the maximum number of hours you will work per week?

Examples:

1. I will return to my job and will not work over 45 hours in a week.
2. I will begin looking for a job in one week. I will apply to at least two places per week.
3. I will quit my bartending job immediately.

9. **Legal Issues:** Include court dates and planning.

Examples:

1. I will attend my DWI hearing on _________.
2. I have an appointment with my lawyer on _________.
3. I have no legal issues pending.

10. **Family Relationships:** Include a plan for activities with family members **and** a plan for dealing with using family members.

Examples:

1. I will go out to dinner or to a movie with my wife once a week.
2. I will plan an activity with my children once a week on Saturdays.
3. I will call my brother and tell him I cannot have drinking in my house when he comes to visit.
4. I will not attend my cousin's wedding next week since there will be alcohol there.

11. **Social Growth:** This is a plan for developing sober relationships and for detaching from using ones. What will you do to make sober friends?

Examples:

1. I will call John from my treatment group two times a week.
2. I will go out for coffee with my sponsor one time a week.
3. I will go to the AA sober dance in two weeks.
4. I will go the AA conference in Albuquerque in September.
5. I will contact my friend, Boozer and tell him that I quit using, and that I won't be around anymore (or when he is drinking).

12. **Leisure Time:** What will you do for fun? What interests or hobbies do you plan on resuming now that you are sober?

Examples:

1. I will go fishing at least once a month.
2. I will attend pottery classes one time per week.
3. I will hike every two weeks with a friend.
4. I will practice my guitar twice a week for one hour.

13. Fire Drill: This is your action plan for when you feel like drinking.

Example:

1. I will call my sponsor.
2. I will double up my meetings for three days and talk about my craving.
3. I will read The Big Book.
4. I will talk about it with my wife/husband.
5. I will read my Step One.

14. Relapse Plan: If I use, what can I do **now** to keep me in recovery?

Examples:

1. Call my sponsor or a friend in AA if my sponsor is not available.
2. Tell my family within 24 hours.
3. Restart 90 meetings in 90 days.
4. Tell my Aftercare Group.

The shame of relapse can keep you using. It will only get smaller if you let someone know what happened.

Name ____________________

Date ____________________

RECOVERY PLAN

1. Remaining chemically free:

2. Meetings:

DAY	TIME	LOCATION
Sunday		
Monday		
Tuesday		
Wednesday		
Thursday		
Friday		
Saturday		

3. Sponsorship:

4. Working The Steps:

5. Spiritual Practice:

6. Physical Health:

7. Emotional Health:

The emotion that places me at greatest risk for reactive behavior is:

When I feel_____________, I will:

a.

b.

c.

8. Employment:

9. Legal Issues:

10. Family Relationships:

11. Social Growth:

12. Leisure Activities:

13. Fire Drill: Five things I will do if I want to use:

a.

b.

c.

d.

e.

14. Relapse Plan: Things that I will do if I relapse:

a.

b.

c.

d.

e.

BIBLIOGRAPHY

Alcoholics Anonymous.

Al-Anon.

Beattie, Melody, *Facing Codependence,* San Francisco: Harper, 1989.

Beattie, Melody, *Codependent No More,* Center City, Minnesota: Hazelden, 1987.

Beattie, Melody, *Beyond Codependency,* San Francisco: Harper/Hazelden, 1989.

Becker, Robert PhD., *Addicted to Misery, The Other Side of Codependency,* Deerfield, Fl: Health Communications, Inc., 1989.

Bepco, Claudia with JoAnn Krestan, *The Responsibility Trap,* New York: The Free Press, 1985.

Black, Claudia, *It Will Never Happen To Me,* New York: Ballantine Books, 1981.

Blatner, Adam, M.D., *Foundations Of Psychodrama,* New York: Springer, 1988.

Bradshaw, John, *Healing The Shame That Binds You,* Deerfield Beach, Fl: Health Communications, Inc., 1988.

Dowling, Colette, *The Cinderella Complex - Women's Hidden Fear Of Independence,* New York: Pocket Books, 1981.

Friel, John, and Linda Friel, *Adult Children, The Secrets of Dysfunctional Families ,* Deerfield Beach, Fl: Health Communications, Inc. , 1988.

Gorski, Terence, Merlene Miller, *Counseling For Relapse Prevention,* Independence, Mo: Herald House, 1982.

Johnson, Stephen M., *Humanizing The Narcissistic Style,* New York/London: W.W. Norton & Co., 1987.

Larsen, Ernie, *Stage II Recovery: Life Beyond Addiction,* San Francisco: Harper & Row, 1985.

Mellody, Pia, *Facing Codependence,* San Francisco: Harper, 1989.

Miller, Alice, *For Your Own Good,* New York: Noonday Press, 1990.

Norwood, Robin, *Women Who Love Too Much,* Los Angeles: Jeremy P. Tarcher, 1985.

Ohmns, David M.D., *The Disease Of Alcoholism,* Cahokie, Il: Gary Whiteaker Corp, 1982.

Peck, M. Scott M.D., *The Road Less Traveled,* New York: Simon and Schuster, 1978.

Rubin, Theodore, The Angry Book, New York: MacMillan, 1970.

Schaeff, Ann Wilson, Codependence, Misunderstood - Mistreated, San Francisco: Harper & Row, 1986.

Stettbacher, J Konrad, Making Sense Of Suffering,. New York: Dutton, 1991.

Subby, Robert, Lost In The Shuffle: The Codependent Reality, Pompano, Fl: Health Communications, Inc., 1987.

Wegscheider-Cruse, Sharon, The Miracle Of Recovery, Deerfield, Fl: Health Communications, Inc., 1989.

Woititz, Janet Geringer Ed,D., Adult Children Of Alcoholics, Hollywood, Fl: Health Communications, Inc., 1983.

U.S. Dept. Of Health And Human Services, Alcohol And Health, Rockville, Md: Public Health Service, 1990.

TO ORDER :

Cost per Manual = $130.00
(20% Discount for 2 or more, = $104.00 ea.)
NM Residents add 6.125% Sales Tax = $7.96

Shipping & Handling = $8.00
(Allow 4-6 weeks)

Telephone Orders : 1-800-203-3597 Monday - Friday 8:30 - 5:30 Mountain Standard Time
Visa & Master Card accepted.

Hospital Purchase Orders : Please include the Purchase Order number, the "ship to" and "bill to" addresses.
Our payment terms are net 30 days.

Postal Orders : Send to:

CL Productions
342 Hillside Ave
Santa Fe, NM 87501

Please Include :

Name ______________________________

Dept ______________________________

Institution ______________________________

Address ______________________________

Tel. # ______________________________

TO ORDER :

Cost per Manual = $130.00

(20% Discount for 2 or more, = $104.00 ea.)
NM Residents add 6.125% Sales Tax = $7.96

Shipping & Handling = $8.00

(Allow 4-6 weeks)

Telephone Orders : 1-800-203-3597 Monday - Friday 8:30 - 5:30 Mountain Standard Time
Visa & Master Card accepted.

Hospital Purchase Orders : Please include the Purchase Order number, the "ship to" and "bill to" addresses.
Our payment terms are net 30 days.

Postal Orders : Send to:

CL Productions
342 Hillside Ave
Santa Fe, NM 87501

Please Include :

Name ______________________________

Dept ______________________________

Institution ______________________________

Address ______________________________

Tel. # ______________________________